365 Tasty Fish Recipes

(365 Tasty Fish Recipes - Volume 1)

Jennifer Wilson

Published on November, 19 2020

Content

365 Awesome Fish Recipes

***

1. 1st Place Baked Salmon Recipe

Serving: 6 | Prep: | Cook: 15mins | Ready in:

Ingredients

- 6 4-oz salmon fillets, each 1 in. thick
- 1 Tablespoon olive oil
- Splash lemon juice(enough to moisten each fillet)
- Fresh rosemary to taste
- paprika to taste
- adobo seasoning to taste
- black pepper to taste
- salt to taste
- honey to taste
- 1/4 Cup chopped pecans
- Non-stick cooking spray

Direction

- Preheat oven to 450 degrees F. In oven, preheat baking dish drizzled with olive oil.
- Place fillets skin-side down on flat surface, rub with lemon juice.
- Sprinkle with seasonings in following order:
- Rosemary - paprika - adobo - black pepper - and salt.
- Lightly drizzle with honey; sprinkle with pecans and seal with generous coating of cooking spray.
- Place fillets skin-side down in preheated baking dish.
- Bake 10 - 15 minutes or until fillets flake easily with fork.
- Serves 6
- Exchanges: 3 meats, 1/2 fat

2. Alaskan Apple Spiced Halibut Or Salmon Recipe

Serving: 8 | Prep: | Cook: 45mins | Ready in:

Ingredients

- 8 (12 oz) halibut fillets or salmon fillets
- 1 shallot, diced (about 1/4 cup)
- 1/4 cup apple jelly
- 1 Tbsp lemon juice
- 1/2 tsp allspice
- 3 Tbsp slivered almonds
- 2 Tbsp butter, melted

Direction

- Preheat oven to 325 degrees F.
- In a small saucepan, heat the apple jelly until liquid. Add the lemon juice and allspice, then stir well.
- Place the halibut fillets in a lightly-buttered baking dish, then brush the glaze over them.
- Add the melted butter to the baking dish and pour the remaining glaze over the fillets, Sprinkle with shallot and almonds.
- Cover pan and bake at 325 degrees F for 10 minutes for every 1 inch of fillet thickness (probably between 35-45 minutes), spooning the glaze periodically over the fillets as they bake.
- Serve with a nice pilaf and vegetable (buttered French cut green beans are good).

3. Angel Hair Pasta With Smoked Salmon And Dill Dated 1966 Recipe

Serving: 6 | Prep: | Cook: 30mins | Ready in:

Ingredients

- 6 ounces angel hair pasta
- 1/2 cup whipping cream
- 1/2 cup milk
- 1/4 cup chopped fresh dill
- 1/4 cup chopped green onions
- 1-1/2 tablespoons drained capers
- 1 teaspoon grated lemon peel
- 4 ounces thinly sliced smoked salmon cut into thin strips

Direction

- Cook pasta in large pot of boiling salted water until just tender but still firm to bite.
- Drain well then return to same pot.
- Combine cream, milk, dill, onions, capers and lemon peel in heavy small saucepan.
- Bring to boil over medium high heat.
- Add sauce to pasta then toss to coat.
- Add salmon and toss to combine then season with salt and pepper and serve.

4. Apple Cider Cured Smoked Salmon Recipe

Serving: 4 | Prep: | Cook: 25mins | Ready in:

Ingredients

- 1 cup brown sugar
- 1/4 cup salt
- 4 cups apple cider or juice
- 2 cinnamon sticks
- 1 teaspoon fennel seeds
- 1 teaspoon whole allspice
- 1 teaspoon black peppercorns
- 1 bay leaf
- 1 teaspoon red pepper flakes
- 6 sprigs thyme or 1/2 teaspoon dried thyme
- 1 large salmon fillets (about 1 pound each), skin and pin bones removed
- A small bundle of wood chips or chunks

Direction

- To make the brine: In a saucepan, combine the brown sugar, salt, and apple juice and bring to a boil. Add the remaining brine ingredients, remove from the heat, and cool. This brine can be made 2 to 3 days in advance and kept in the refrigerator.
- Submerge the salmon fillets in the liquid brine for at least 6 hours or overnight, refrigerated. Remove the salmon from the brine and place, uncovered, on a wire rack set in a sheet pan. Refrigerate the fillets for at least 6 hours, or overnight, to dry them out. (A dry fillet will take on smoke quicker than a moist fillet)
- To smoke the salmon: In an outdoor grill, make a small fire using mesquite charcoal or briquettes. Once the fire has burned down to a hot bed of coals, after about 1 hour, place the soaked wood on the coals. Position the grate 8 to 12 inches above the smoking wood and place the salmon fillets on the grate.
- Cover the grill and shut any open-air vents. After 5 minutes, check the heat of the grill; large fillets will be cooked and smoked through in approximately 30 minutes if the heat is low, about 300 to 350 degrees F, while a hotter fire will cook the fillets in 15 to 20 minutes. Serve the salmon hot off the grill.

5. Apricot Ginger Glazed Salmon Recipe

Serving: 4 | Prep: | Cook: 15mins | Ready in:

Ingredients

- 1 pound wild salmon fillet (copper river is the best!)
- salt and freshly ground black pepper
- 3 tablespoons apricot jam or preserves
- 3 teaspoons grated fresh ginger
- 2 teaspoons soy sauce
- 1/2 teaspoon crushed red pepper (optional)

Direction

- Preheat oven to 450°F.
- Cut fillets into equal servings. Pat salmon dry and season with salt and pepper; place skin side down on greased or parchment-lined (for easy clean up) rimmed baking sheet.
- In small bowl, stir together jam, ginger and soy sauce - and red pepper if you want to add some spicy-hot to it. Spread evenly over salmon.
- Roast 10 to 15 minutes, or until salmon flakes easily. The glaze may caramelize a bit.

6. Asiago Herb Encrusted Salmon Recipe

Serving: 8 | Prep: | Cook: 10mins | Ready in:

Ingredients

- 2/3 cup dry, unseasoned breadcrumbs
- 1/4 cup grated asiago cheese
- 2 sprigs fresh rosemary
- 1/2 tbsp garlic powder
- 1 tbsp dried basil
- 1/2 tsp black pepper
- 1 egg, beaten with
- 1/4 cup buttermilk
- 1 1/2 lb sockeye salmon, cut into 8 equal pieces
- 2 tsp olive oil

Direction

- Combine breadcrumbs through pepper in a shallow dish.
- Pour egg and buttermilk mixture into another shallow dish.
- Dip each salmon piece into buttermilk mixture, then coat completely in breadcrumb mix, pressing it onto the fish, and set onto a plate.
- Cover and refrigerate 30 minutes - 1 hour.
- Heat oil in a non-stick fry pan over medium heat.
- Add fish in one layer and cook 5 minutes per side.

7. Asian Salmon Fillets Recipe

Serving: 2 | Prep: | Cook: 35mins | Ready in:

Ingredients

- 1/4 lb. slice of salmon per person
- butter
- garlic powder
- powdered ginger
- ground pepper
- orange juice
- soy sauce

Direction

- Grease a baking dish with butter
- Place the salmon skin-side down in it
- Sprinkle with the garlic powder, ginger, and freshly ground pepper.
- Sprinkle some soy sauce over the fish and then pour orange juice in, about 1/2 inch deep.
- Dot the top of the fish with butter.
- Cover and microwave on high if making two or three servings. For two servings I nuke this 3 1/2 minutes. If preparing for numerous people I'd cook on a lower power and adjust the time so the fish doesn't explode.

8. Baked Alaskan Halibut Supreme Recipe

Serving: 7 | Prep: | Cook: 30mins | Ready in:

Ingredients

- cooking spray
- 3 lb halibut fillet(s)
- butter
- salt
- pepper
- 1/2 cup parmesan cheese
- 4-6 strips of bacon
- 1 tsp lemon juice
- 1 cup sour cream
- 1/3 cup buttered bread crumbs (3T butter, melted + 1/3 cup Crumbs)
- chopped parsley

Direction

- Rub halibut with butter, salt and pepper.
- Spray baking pan with cooking spray.
- Lay bacon on the bottom of baking pan and place fillet(s) on top.
- Make a mixture of sour cream, cheese, crumbs, and lemon juice.
- Spread over the fish.
- Bake at 350 until tender (20-30 minutes)
- Serve with grated cheese and parsley!!

9. Baked Fish With Vegetables Recipe

Serving: 4 | Prep: | Cook: 60mins | Ready in:

Ingredients

- 4 lbs. fish (whitefish, carp or salmon trout)
- 1 T. salt
- 1/2 t. garlic salt
- 1 t. paprika
- 1 large onion
- 1 green pepper
- 2 stalks celery
- 2 carrots
- 3 Ts. melted butter or oil
- 1/2 c. sour cream
- 1 c. green peas
- 2 medium potatoes

Direction

- Mix seasoning. Clean fish, rub in seasoning and let stand until ready for oven. Place onion, celery, green pepper and oil in a baking dish in moderate, 350°, oven until slightly sautéed. Arrange fish in baking dish, cover with sautéed mixture and bake for 1/2 hour. Cut carrots and potatoes into small chunks and scatter into baking dish. Add the green peas and bake for another 1/2hour, or until fish is done. About ten minutes before turning off oven, when fish is nearly done, pour the sour cream over the fish and let stand in hot oven.

10. Baked Flounder With Minced Clams Recipe

Serving: 4 | Prep: | Cook: 25mins | Ready in:

Ingredients

- 1 1/2 lbs. flounder fillets
- 1 onion, finely minced
- 1 c. dry white wine
- 1 1/2 TB flour
- 2 TB butter, melted
- 1 c. hot cooking liquid
- 1/2 c. heavy cream
- 1 (8oz.) can minced clams, drained

Direction

- Arrange fillets in a shallow baking dish; add minced onion and dry white wine. Bake the fillets in a preheated 325° oven until they are just done or for 15 to 20 minutes.

- Transfer the fillets carefully to a heatproof serving dish and keep them warm. Reserve 1 c. cooking liquid.
- Make a sauce with the flour blended with melted butter. Gradually add the 1 cup of hot cooking liquid. Simmer the sauce, stirring often, until it is smooth and thickened, then, add heavy cream and minced clams. Taste the sauce for seasoning, stir it until it is hot but not boiling, and pour it over the fish fillets.
- Put the dish under a broiler for a few minutes until the sauce bubbles and begins to glaze. Serve while hot.

11. Baked Haddock Almondine Recipe

Serving: 2 | Prep: | Cook: 20mins | Ready in:

Ingredients

- 1 cup coarsely ground dry bread crumbs
- 1/4 cup toasted sliced almonds
- 3 tablespoons butter melted
- 1 teaspoon kosher salt
- 2 skinless haddock fillets
- 1/4 cup all-purpose flour
- 2/3 cup mayonnaise
- 1-1/2 cups water

Direction

- Preheat oven to 350.
- In a small bowl combine crumbs, almonds, butter and salt.
- Mix well.
- If necessary, add extra butter to hold crumbs together.
- Coat fish with flour, shaking off excess.
- Place fillets in a baking pan large enough to hold them in a single layer.
- Spread mayonnaise over the entire surface of fish.
- Cover evenly with crumb mixture lightly pressing into the fish.
- Carefully pour water around the fish.
- Bake for 20 minutes.

12. Baked Haddock Recipe

Serving: 4 | Prep: | Cook: 15mins | Ready in:

Ingredients

- 4 haddock fillets
- 3/4c milk
- 2tsp. salt
- 3/4c bread crumbs
- 1/4c grated parmesan cheese
- 1/4tsp ground thyme
- 1/4c melted butter

Direction

- Preheat oven to 500. In a small bowl, mix milk and salt. In separate bowl, mix bread crumbs, parmesan cheese, and thyme. Dip haddock in milk, press crumb mix into fillets to coat. Place fillets in a glass baking dish, drizzle with melted butter. Bake top rack for 15 minutes.

13. Baked Haddock With Lime And Tomato Sauce Recipe

Serving: 4 | Prep: | Cook: 25mins | Ready in:

Ingredients

- 4 haddock fillets skinned and boned
- Sauce:
- 3 tablespoons vegetable oil
- 2 medium red onions finely chopped
- 1-1/2 teaspoons ground coriander
- 1/2 teaspoon cayenne
- 1 red bell pepper diced
- 1 green bell pepper diced
- 4 tomatoes peeled seeded and diced

- 6 tablespoons lime juice
- 1/2 teaspoon salt
- 1 teaspoon freshly ground black pepper
- 2 tablespoons chopped fresh cilantro

Direction

- Preheat oven to 375 degrees.
- Rinse fillets and pat dry.
- In large saucepan heat oil over medium high heat.
- Add onions and cook until tender about 10 minutes.
- Stir in coriander and cayenne then cook 2 minutes.
- Add diced red and green peppers and tomatoes.
- Reduce heat to low and cook uncovered for 10 minutes.
- Remove saucepan from heat and stir in lime juice then season with salt and pepper.
- Arrange fillets in a buttered shallow baking dish then cover with sauce.
- Bake uncovered for 25 minutes then sprinkle with cilantro and serve.

14. Baked Halibut Recipe

Serving: 6 | Prep: | Cook: 30mins | Ready in:

Ingredients

- 3 lbs. halibut fillet, cut into 6 serving pieces, 3/4 inch thick
- 1/4 cup minced fresh parsley
- 1/2 cup seasoned bread crumbs
- 2 lemons, sliced, plus 2 more thinly sliced for garnish
- 2 Tbsp lemon cello liquor
- 1 tsp paprika
- 2 cloves garlic, minced
- 1 Tbsp butter
- salt and pepper to taste

Direction

- Preheat oven to 375 degrees.
- Sprinkle both sides of fish with salt and pepper and paprika.
- Place fish in a buttered shallow baking dish and sprinkle with garlic, parsley and breadcrumbs.
- Place lemon slices on fish, lemon cello, and add water almost to top of fish.
- Bake uncovered 20-30 minutes until fish is firm and crumbs are golden brown.
- Remove lemon slices, dot with butter and place under broiler until browned.
- Garnish with thin lemon slices.

15. Baked Paprika Flounder Recipe

Serving: 4 | Prep: | Cook: 10mins | Ready in:

Ingredients

- 4 to 5 small flounder filets
- butter cooking spray
- salt
- pepper
- Italian herbs
- paprika

Direction

- Preheat oven to 400 degrees.
- Spray baking sheet with cooking spray. Place filets on baking sheet and spray them lightly.
- Sprinkle coarse salt, ground pepper, Italian herbs and paprika to taste. It's good with a lot of paprika.
- Bake at 400 degrees for ten minutes or until white and flaky.

16. Baked Salmon Stuffed With Spinach Cream Cheese Recipe

Serving: 2 | Prep: | Cook: 12mins | Ready in:

Ingredients

- 2-3 oz. fresh spinach, chopped
- 1/4 cup cream cheese, room temperature
- Pinch of nutmeg
- salt and pepper
- 2 (6-8 oz.) salmon fillets about 1-inch thick, with skin on
- olive oil
- 3/4 cup fresh breadcrumbs from a crusty Italian-style bread
- 4 TB. melted butter
- 1/4 cup grated parmesan cheese

Direction

- Put spinach in a small saucepan with 1 TB. of water.
- Cook 1-2 minutes just to wilt the spinach. Rinse with cold water and squeeze dry.
- Combine spinach with cream cheese and nutmeg. Season with salt and pepper.
- Cut a 1/2-inch deep slit in the middle of each salmon fillet, with skin side down.
- From the bottom of the slit, cut the fillet horizontally about 1-inch in both directions to form a pocket for the stuffing.
- Fill with the cream cheese mixture.
- Preheat oven to 450 degrees F.
- Brush a baking sheet with olive oil.
- Sprinkle salmon with salt and pepper.
- Combine breadcrumbs, butter and Parmesan cheese.
- Top each fillet with the crumbs, covering each top and pressing to adhere.
- Place salmon on baking sheet.
- Bake 12 minutes or until fish is opaque. Serve with grilled vegetables, if desired.

17. Baked Salmon Stuffed And Wrapped In Grape Vine Leaves Recipe

Serving: 6 | Prep: | Cook: 35mins | Ready in:

Ingredients

- 800g salmon in one piece (not tail end)
- 10-12 preserved grape vine leaves
- 1 small fennel bulb
- 3 tblspns roasted pine nuts (preroast for 10 mins at 180 deg C)
- 1/4 cup currants, reconstituted in verjuice
- 3 x 1/4 preserved lemons, skin only, sliced thinly
- 1/2 red (spanish) onion, small dice
- 1 tblspn chopped chervil
- 2 tblspns fennel leaves (from top of bulb used in baking)
- 50g butter
- 1/4 cup verjuice

Direction

- OVERNIGHT
- Reconstitute the currants in verjuice.
- Roast the pine nuts and allow to cool.
- COOKING DAY
- Preheat oven to 120 deg C.
- Slice the base of the fennel bulb and spread over a small baking tray (reserve the top for garnish).
- Cut the salmon into two equal pieces.
- Make a stuffing by mixing together the roasted pine nuts, currants, finely chopped onion, herbs and 25g of butter to hold it together.
- Rinse the grape leaves, pat dry and lay out on a fresh chopping board for the 'salmon sandwich'.
- Place one piece of salmon down and season well with salt and pepper.
- Place all stuffing on top.
- Place second piece of salmon on top of the stuffing mix and season well.
- Wrap the parcel in the vine leaves and tie with string, making sure the leaves are covering all the salmon.
- Place this parcel on top of the sliced fennel, add verjuice/white wine and the rest of the butter.
- Bake at 120 deg C for 50 minutes, turning once after 25-30 mins.

- Baste with pan juices once or twice through cooking.
- Notes:
- At the finish of cooking time, take salmon parcel from the oven and allow to rest for 10 mins upside down.
- Turn oven up to 200 deg C to finish cooking the fennel.
- Return the rested salmon parcel to the oven to 'flash' reheat before cutting off the string and carving into thick slices.
- Garnish with the fennel tops and a spray of chervil along with a verjuice beurre blanc.

18. Baked Sea Bass With Rosemary And Garlic Recipe

Serving: 4 | Prep: | Cook: 15mins | Ready in:

Ingredients

- 1 large sea bass, about 1kg, scaled and gutted
- rosemary sprigs
- about 2 garlic clove thinly sliced
- lemon slices
- lemon juice
- small bunch basil leaves
- olive oil
- sea salt
- foil

Direction

- Preheat oven to 200C / gas 6.
- Stuff the cavity with lemon and some of the rosemary.
- Lay the fish on an oiled, foil-covered baking tray.
- Make about 6 slashes down its side.
- First lay the basil leaves over the slashes.
- Then poke the rosemary and garlic slices into the slashes.
- Drizzle with olive oil and sprinkle with sea salt and lemon juice.
- Bake for about 15 -20 mins.
- When fin pulls out easily then it's done.

19. Baked Stuffed Tilapia Recipe

Serving: 8 | Prep: | Cook: 30mins | Ready in:

Ingredients

- 16 small to medium tilapia fillets, aim for the same size; you are making a tilapia sandwich with the stuffing.
- salt and pepper for sprinkling
- juice of three lemons, divided use
- 10 slices of white bread, toasted and cubed
- 1/2 teaspoon of dry mustard
- 1/2 teaspoon of dried dill weed
- 4 tablespoons of minced shallots
- 1 tablespoon of dry white vermouth
- 1 can of artichoke hearts, drained and chopped
- 1 cup of chicken broth more or less as needed
- 1 refrigerator can of crabmeat (cheapest, not fancy; you're mixing it in a stuffing here) drained
- 1 cup of butter, melted divided use
- 1 egg yolk
- 1/2 cup of heavy cream, whipped to soft peaks
- 1/8 teaspoon of salt
- 1/4 cup of parmesan cheese
- 1/4 cup of toasted bread crumbs

Direction

- Preheat oven to 350 degrees.
- Line a sheet pan with foil (you want something with sides here).
- Lightly grease the foil (I use my butter wrappers for this).
- Lay 8 of the tilapia fillets on the baking sheet.
- Sprinkle lightly with salt and pepper and a squeeze of lemon juice.
- In a large bowl, combine bread cubes, shallots dill, mustard, vermouth, artichokes and crabmeat.

- Add 1/2 cup of melted butter and enough chicken broth to moisten. You want it to hold together and not fall apart here.
- Top each tilapia with a scoop of filling, flatten slightly.
- Top with remaining tilapia fillet (match up sizes if you can).
- Sprinkle with more salt and pepper and some more dill.
- Cover with foil tent. Bake in oven for 15 minutes.
- While fish is in oven, make glaze. Beat yolk and salt until foamy.
- Gradually add in 2 tablespoons of melted butter.
- Mix remaining butter with 2 teaspoons of lemon juice and add to the egg yolk mixture. Fold in the whipped cream.
- Pull stuffed fish out of oven, remove foil.
- Turn oven to broil. Spoon a generous spoon of glaze over each fish piece. Sprinkle with bread crumbs and parmesan cheese.
- Broil until golden brown and toasted.
- "Fish, to taste right, must swim three times - in water, in butter, and in wine."
- Polish proverb

20. Baked Tilapia With Garlic Lime And Cilantro Recipe

Serving: 4 | Prep: | Cook: 25mins | Ready in:

Ingredients

- ½ cup lime juice
- 1 to 2 tbsp extra virgin olive oil
- 2 to 3 garlic cloves, peeled and minced
- 1 to 2 fresh jalapeno peppers, chopped, seeds removed, if desired
- 1 tablespoon finely snipped fresh cilantro leaves or 1 teaspoon dried cilantro
- 1 to 2 tsp. grated fresh lime peel (optional)
- 1 teaspoon honey (optional)
- salt and cayenne pepper to taste
- 1½ to 2 pounds tilapia fillets or other mild white fish fillets
- 1 to 2 chopped firm ripe tomatoes (optional)
- paprika and thin lime slices for garnish (optional)

Direction

- In a deep medium glass or ceramic bowl, combine all ingredients except fish fillets tomatoes and garnish, blending well.
- Arrange fish fillets in the marinade, coating each piece well.
- Cover with plastic wrap and refrigerate for about 1 hour, turning fish fillets occasionally. Drain off marinade, reserving marinade for basting fish.
- Arrange fish fillets in a baking dish.
- Baste fillets liberally with marinade.
- Top with tomatoes if using.
- Bake, loosely covered with aluminum foil, in a preheated moderate oven (350'F.) for 20 to 25 minutes or until fillets are opaque in color and flake easily with a fork, basting occasionally with marinade.
- Garnish with a sprinkle and thin slices of lime if desired.

21. Baked White Fish With Onions Peppers Olives And Feta Recipe

Serving: 2 | Prep: | Cook: 20mins | Ready in:

Ingredients

- 2 or 3 medium-sized Tilapia filets
- (for best results, use fish that is uniformly thick)
- 1/2 T olive oil (or less, depending on your pan)
- 1/2 cup very finely diced red pepper
- 1/4 cup of sliced pepperoncini peppers
- 1/4 cup very finely diced red onion (or sweet white onion)
- 1/4 cup very finely diced green olives

- 1/3 cup crumbled feta (or less if you're not wild about feta)
- 1-2 T mayo

Direction

- Preheat oven to 425. Spray small glass or ceramic casserole dish with nonstick spray.
- Heat olive oil in nonstick frying pan and sauté red pepper and onion about 3 minutes. Add olives and sauté about 2 minutes more. Turn off heat.
- Put fish in casserole dish and season with salt and pepper. Spread a small amount of mayo evenly over the surface of each piece of fish.
- Stir feta into red pepper/pepperoncini/onion/olive mixture and spread that over the top of fish. (Pile it on so all the mixture is used. It doesn't matter if some falls off while it's cooking.)
- Bake until fish is opaque and white throughout and topping is barely starting to brown, 10-15 minutes.
- The mayo and the topping will keep the fish moist. Serve hot.

22. Barbeque Salmon Steaks Recipe

Serving: 4 | Prep: | Cook: 20mins | Ready in:

Ingredients

- 4 salmon steaks
- 3 tablespoons melted butter
- 1 tablespoon fresh lemon juice
- 1 tablespoon white wine vinegar
- 1/4 teaspoon grated lemon peel
- 1/4 teaspoon garlic salt
- 1/4 teaspoon salt
- 1 teaspoon hot pepper sauce

Direction

- Combine all ingredients except salmon stirring thoroughly.
- Generously brush both sides of salmon steaks with mixture.
- Barbeque on a well-oiled grill over hot coals.
- Make a tent of foil or use barbeque cover and place over salmon.
- Barbeque for 8 minutes per side depending.
- Baste frequently turning once brushing with sauce.

23. Battered Flounder Bites Recipe

Serving: 10 | Prep: | Cook: 15mins | Ready in:

Ingredients

- Sauce:
- 1 cup mayo
- 2 Tbs chopped shallots
- 1 tbs chopped jalepeno peppers
- 2 tsp hot sauce
- 1 tsp lemon juice
- 1/4 tsp salt
- dash red pepper flakes
- Fish:
- 1, 8 oz pkg hush puppy mix
- 3/4 cup milk
- 1 1/4 lb flounder fillets cut into 1/2 inch pieces
- 2 cups of oil to fry
- 1 cup flour to dredge fish

Direction

- Combine sauce ingredients and cover and chill.
- Prepare fish:
- Heat oil to 350F.
- Combine hushpuppy mix and milk into a batter.
- Dip fish into flour and then into batter.
- Fry golden about 3 to 4 minutes per side.
- Serve with sauce.

24. Bbq Salmon With Roasted Corn Amp Black Bean Salsa Recipe

Serving: 4 | Prep: | Cook: 8mins | Ready in:

Ingredients

- 4 salmon Filets, 6 to 8 oz. each
- kosher salt & fresh ground pepper
- extra virgin olive oil for searing
- ½ cup honey-Citrus BBQ Sauce
- FOR THE salsa
- 1 cup canned black beans, drained & rinsed
- 1/4 cup chopped cilantro
- 1 cup roasted corn, removed from cob
- 1/2 cup lime juice
- 1/2 medium red onion, diced
- 1/4 cup olive oil
- 1/2 medium red bell pepper, diced
- 1/2 tablespoon ground cumin
- 1/2 medium poblano pepper, diced
- 1/2 tablespoon black pepper
- 1/2 cup seeded diced tomato
- 1 tablespoon salt
- SWEET AND SMOKEY BBQ SAUCE
- 1/3 cup apple cider vinegar
- 1 cup ketchup
- 3 tablespoons brown sugar
- 1 tablespoon yellow mustard
- 1 tablespoon molasses
- 2 tablespoon worcestershire sauce
- 1 teaspoon liquid smoke
- juice of 1 orange
- 1 teaspoon salt 1/2 tsp dried crushed red pepper
- 1 tsp hot sauce
- 1 tsp soy sauce

Direction

- SALSA DIRECTIONS
- Combine all ingredients in a large bowl up to and including the cilantro
- In a separate bowl, add the lime juice and spices, whisk in the olive oil a little at a time. Add to the salsa and toss gently to combine. Refrigerate for at least one hour.
- SALMON COOKING DIRECTIONS
- Preheat oven to 425 degrees.
- Pre-heat skillet over medium heat, (I like to use a good quality non-stick skillet for the first part of this process, but a cast iron skillet or grill pan will also work, or this can also be done on the grill.)
- Salt & pepper both sides of the salmon filets and drizzle some olive oil in the pan.
- Sear the filets no more than 3 minutes on each side.
- Carefully transfer the salmon to a foil or parchment lined sheet pan and brush generously with the barbecue sauce on the top and sides of each filet.
- Place the pan in a 425 degree oven for 5 minutes or until the barbecue sauce begins to caramelize.
- Serve over a mound of the roasted corn & black bean salsa and garnish with a few sprigs of fresh cilantro.
- SWEET & SMOKEY BBQ SAUCE DIRECTIONS
- Combine vinegar, liquid smoke, and brown sugar. Stir until sugar is dissolved.
- Add and combine the rest of ingredients well and refrigerate.

25. Beer Battered Fish Fry With Homemade Tartar Sauce Recipe

Serving: 6 | Prep: | Cook: 10mins | Ready in:

Ingredients

- fish
- 2 cups biscuit mix
- 1 teaspoon dried dill weed
- 1/2 teaspoon onion powder
- 1/2 teaspoon garlic powder
- 1/2 teaspoon salt
- 1/2 teaspoon pepper
- 2 cups (16-ounces) beer

- 2 eggs, slightly beaten
- 2 to 3 pounds fish fillets*, cut into serving-size pieces
- Additional biscuit mix
- *halibut, ling cod, salmon, trout, red snapper, bass and catfish do very nicely
- tartar sauce
- (I have never measured this in my life! Do a taste test and adjust if needed - I think this should be right)
- 1/3 c Dukes Real Mayo
- 1 -2 t minced onion (white or green)
- 2 t dill relish (sold by the pickles, it's just minced dill pickles)
- juice from a lemon wedge

Direction

- FISH
- In a large mixing bowl, combine mix, dill weed, onion powder, garlic powder, salt and pepper together.
- Add beer and eggs and mix well.
- Dredge fish fillets in additional biscuit mix and immerse in the prepared batter.
- Refrigerate fillets in the batter for 20 to 30 minutes.
- Heat deep-fat fryer to 375*F (190*C).
- Remove fillets from the batter one at a time, allowing excess batter to drip off.
- Fry 2 to 3 fillets at a time in the hot oil until golden brown, about 3 to 5 minutes.
- (Over-crowding will result in reduced temperature of the oil causing the fish to absorb the oil and become greasy.)
- Drain on paper towels.
- TATAR SAUCE
- Stir together and serve with hot fish

26. Beer Battered Fish With Smoked Paprika Mayonnaise Recipe

Serving: 4 | Prep: | Cook: 15mins | Ready in:

Ingredients

- 6 to 8 cups vegetable oil for frying
- 3/4 cup all-purpose flour
- 3/4 teaspoon salt
- 3/4 cup beer (not dark)
- 8 (2 1/2-oz) pieces of pollack, Pacific cod, or catfish fillet (3/4 to 1 inch thick)
- 1/4 cup drained bottled capers, coarsely chopped
- 3/4 teaspoon hot Spanish smoked paprika
- 1/2 cup mayonnaise
- ****
- Special equipment: a deep-fat thermometer
- Garnish: lemon wedges

Direction

- Heat 2 inches oil in a wide 5- to 6-quart heavy pot over high heat until it registers 380°F on thermometer.
- While oil is heating, whisk together flour and salt in a shallow bowl, then whisk in beer (batter will be thick).
- Coat each piece of fish with batter and transfer to hot oil with tongs (remove thermometer). Cook over high heat, turning over once, until golden and just cooked through, 5 to 6 minutes total, then transfer fish to paper towels to drain.
- While fish fries, whisk capers and paprika into mayonnaise in a bowl. Serve with fish.
- Enjoy...yum!

27. Big Ray's Greek Grilled Catfish Recipe

Serving: 8 | Prep: | Cook: 10mins | Ready in:

Ingredients

- 6 (8 ounce) fillets catfish
- 1 tablespoon Greek seasoning, or to taste
- 4 ounces crumbled feta cheese
- 6 toothpicks

- 1 tablespoon dried mint
- 2 tablespoons olive oil

Direction

- Preheat grill for medium heat and lightly oil the grate.
- Season both sides of each catfish fillet with Greek seasoning. Sprinkle feta cheese and mint over one side of each fillet; drizzle olive oil over the cheese and mint. Beginning with narrower end, roll fish tightly around the filling and secure with a toothpick.
- Cook on preheated grill until the fish flakes easily with a fork, 20 to 25 minutes.

28. Blackened Tilapia Recipe

Serving: 4 | Prep: | Cook: 5mins | Ready in:

Ingredients

- 4-6 Tilapia
- 2 Tablespoons - paprika
- 2 Teaspoons - salt (or to taste) **Read recipe alteration below.**
- 2 Teaspoons - lemon pepper
- 1-1/2 Teaspoon - garlic powder
- 1-1/2 Teaspoon - ground red pepper
- 1-1/2 Teaspoon - Dried, Crushed basil
- 1 Teaspoon - onion powder
- 1 Teaspoon - Dried thyme
- 1 Cup - unsalted butter, melted (I always start with a stick of butter melted and then melt more if needed.)

Direction

- Heat iron skillet on high 5 minutes.
- Mix all seasonings in a bowl.
- Dip fillets in melted butter and coat with seasonings. (I drizzle the spices on each piece of fish to get an even coating. Don't be afraid to coat heavily)!!
- Place fillets in hot skillet and cook 2 minutes on each side.
- Makes 4 servings.
- Enjoy!!!

29. Blackened Tuna With Soy Mustard Sauce Recipe

Serving: 2 | Prep: | Cook: 20mins | Ready in:

Ingredients

- 1/4 cup mustard powder
- 2 tablespoons hot water
- 2 tablespoons unseasoned rice vinegar
- 1/4 cup soy sauce
- 1/2 cup white wine
- 2 teaspoons white wine vinegar
- 1 teaspoon fresh lemon juice
- 1 tablespoon minced shallot
- 2 tablespoons heavy cream
- 1/2 cup unsalted butter chopped
- 1/2 teaspoon salt
- 1 teaspoon freshly ground white pepper
- 1-1/2 tablespoons paprika
- 1/2 tablespoon cayenne powder
- 1/2 tablespoon red chile powder
- 1/4 teaspoon freshly ground white pepper
- 8 ounce tuna fillet
- 3 tablespoons red pickled ginger
- 1/2 teaspoon black sesame seeds
- 1 tablespoon cucumber cut into matchsticks

Direction

- Mix mustard powder and hot water together into a paste.
- Let sit a few minutes to allow flavor to develop.
- Add vinegar and soy sauce then mix together and strain through a fine sieve and chill.
- Combine wine, vinegar, juice and shallot in saucepan and bring to boil over medium high heat.

- Reduce liquid until syrupy then add cream and reduce by half.
- Turn heat to low and gradually add butter stirring slowly until incorporated.
- Be careful not to let mixture boil or it will break and separate.
- Season with salt and pepper then strain through a fine sieve.
- Transfer to a double boiler and keep warm.
- Mix all spices together on a plate and dredge tuna on all sides.
- Heat a lightly oiled cast iron skillet and sear tuna over high heat 2 minutes per side.
- Cut into thin slices.
- For each serving arrange 4 slices tuna in a pinwheel or cross shape on the plate.
- Ladle a little soy mustard sauce in two opposing quadrants between the tuna.
- Ladle wine sauce in other two quadrants.
- Put a small mound of pickled ginger over top and sprinkle with sesame seeds and cucumber.

30. Blackened Tilapia Over White Rice With Sauteed Green Beans Recipe

Serving: 2 | Prep: | Cook: 20mins | Ready in:

Ingredients

- 2-4 tilapia fillet pieces
- Zatarans Blackened seasoning
- white rice
- 4tbsp butter/margarine
- 1 can of green beans

Direction

- First, melt 3 tbsp of butter in a saucepan. Once melted, pour into bowl, and coat fish fully in butter. Lay out on pan or foil and season to taste with seasoning (don't be afraid to use a LOT of seasoning). Set fish aside. Boil water for rice, and season to taste. Once water boils and rice is cooking, place left over butter in heavy skillet and heat skillet until hot. Place fish in skillet and cover until fish is flaky. Set rice aside and cover. Remove skillet from heat and remove fish, set aside. Drain can of green beans and place in single layer in skillet. Add 1 tbsp butter, place back on heat and cover. Sauté green beans until hot, and remove from heat. Serve hot.

31. Braised Black Cod With Daikon Radish Recipe

Serving: 6 | Prep: | Cook: 20mins | Ready in:

Ingredients

- Sauce Ingredients:
- 2 cups water
- 1/3 cup soy sauce
- 2 Tbsp red pepper Powder
- 3 garlic cloves, minced
- 2 Pinches ginger powder
- 1/2 daikon radish, peeled and cut into 1/2 inch thick, then cut in 1/2
- Main Ingredients:
- 1 fresh whole cod (about 3 lbs)
- 1 Tbsp sake
- 1 Tbsp corn syrup (Plum Extract:maesilchung or yoridang)
- 1 jalapeno, seeded and sliced
- 1 red pepper, seeded and sliced
- 2 green onions, sliced
- pinch of toasted sesame seed

Direction

- Prepare the sauce - Boil the water in the sauté pan, add soy sauce, ginger, garlic and radish, red pepper powder; boil and reduce heat to medium-low, then cook about 20 minutes.
- In mean time, cut fish into 1 1/2 inch thick and remove the fins with scissors. Cut jalapeno, red pepper and green onions and set aside until the sauce is ready.

- Add fish, Sake, Corn syrup (Maesil Cheong) on top of the sauce mixture. Cook it for about 10 minutes on high-medium. The sauce will start to thicken.
- After 10 minutes, the sauce will be reduced in half. Be careful not to burn it, so keep an eye on it. Also pour the sauce with spoon on the top of the fish so that the fish may absorb the sauce evenly.
- Add 2 chopped green onions, jalapeno and cook for 5 more minutes on high. When it is done, the liquid will be like a thick sauce. This looks absolutely delicious.

32. Braised Orange Roughy With Leeks Recipe

Serving: 4 | Prep: | Cook: 20mins | Ready in:

Ingredients

- 2 tablespoons (1/4 stick) butter
- 3 large leeks (white and pale green parts only), halved lengthwise, sliced
- 2 teaspoons sugar
- 1/2 teaspoon dried thyme, crumbled
- 4 6- to 8-ounce orange roughy fillets (or tilapia)
- 1/2 cup whipping cream (or half and half)
- 1/4 cup dry vermouth (or white wine)
- Fresh chives or green onion tops cut into 1-inch lengths

Direction

- Melt butter in heavy large skillet over medium heat. Add leeks and sprinkle with sugar and thyme. Season with salt and pepper. Sauté 5 minutes. Reduce heat and cover and cook until very soft, stirring occasionally, about 10 minutes. Season fish with salt and pepper. Arrange atop leeks. Add cream and vermouth. Cover and cook until fish is opaque, about 8 minutes. Transfer fish to plates and keep warm.
- Boil sauce until slightly thickened, about 3 minutes. Season to taste with salt and pepper. Top fish with sauce and leeks. Garnish with chives.

33. Braised Sea Bass With Moroccan Spiced Sauce Recipe

Serving: 4 | Prep: | Cook: 20mins | Ready in:

Ingredients

- 1/4 cup chopped coriander
- 1/4 cup chopped parsley
- 3 cloves garlic, chopped
- 2 tbsp olive oil
- 1/2 tsp crushed red pepper flakes or to taste
- 2 tsp ground cumin
- 2 tsp sweet paprika
- Pinch cinnamon
- 3 tbsp lemon juice
- 1 tsp grated lemon zest
- Salt and freshly ground pepper to taste
- Four 6 oz Chilean sea bass fillets, skin removed
- Moroccan spiced Sauce:
- 2 tbsp olive oil
- 1/2 cup chopped onion
- 2 cups chopped canned or fresh tomatoes

Direction

- In a food processor or by hand, combine coriander, parsley and garlic.
- Process until chunky.
- Add olive oil, red pepper flakes, cumin, paprika, cinnamon, lemon juice and zest.
- Season with salt and pepper.
- Process until all ingredients are combined.
- Spread half of spice mixture over fish fillets in a baking dish and marinate for 30 minutes.
- For sauce, heat olive oil in a large skillet on medium heat.

- Add onion and sauté 2 minutes or until onion is softened.
- Stir in remaining spice mixture and tomatoes.
- Simmer together for 10 minutes.
- Place fish on top of sauce, cover and simmer for 10 to 15 minutes or until fish is cooked and it begins to split on top.
- Place fish on serving plate and pour sauce around.

34. Brazilian Fish Stew

Serving: 0 | Prep: | Cook: | Ready in:

Ingredients

- 2 cups water
- 1 cup uncooked white rice
- 1 tablespoon olive oil
- 1 yellow onion, thinly sliced
- 1 teaspoon salt, plus more to taste
- 2 tablespoons tomato paste
- 4 cloves minced garlic
- 2 teaspoons paprika
- 1 teaspoon ground cumin
- cayenne pepper to taste
- 1 (14 ounce) can full-fat coconut milk
- 1 teaspoon soy sauce
- 1 red or yellow bell pepper, halved and thinly sliced
- 2 eaches jalapeno peppers, seeded and thinly sliced
- ¼ cup chopped green onion
- 1 ½ pounds sea bass fillets, cut into chunks
- 1 pinch salt
- ¼ cup chopped cilantro leaves
- 2 tablespoons freshly squeezed lime juice

Direction

- Bring water and rice to a boil in a saucepan. Reduce heat to medium-low, cover, and simmer until rice is tender and liquid has been absorbed, 20 to 25 minutes.
- Heat olive oil in a skillet over medium heat. Add onions and 1 teaspoon salt. Cook and stir just until onions start to get soft, 3 or 4 minutes. Add tomato paste, garlic, paprika, cumin, and cayenne pepper. Continue cooking about 3 minutes. Pour in coconut milk and add soy sauce. When mixture starts to bubble, let it simmer about 5 minutes.
- Increase heat to medium-high. Stir in bell peppers, jalapeno peppers, and green onions. Let mixture come back to a simmer. Transfer fish to skillet; stir. Cover and cook over medium-high heat until fish starts to flake, about 5 minutes. Remove from heat. Add salt, cilantro, and lime juice; stir carefully to avoid breaking up the fish. Serve with rice.
- Nutrition Facts
- Per Serving:
- 399 calories; protein 25.6g 51% DV; carbohydrates 32.6g 11% DV; fat 19g 29% DV; cholesterol 46.9mg 16% DV; sodium 599.8mg 24% DV.

35. Broiled Ginger Albacore Recipe

Serving: 4 | Prep: | Cook: 15mins | Ready in:

Ingredients

- 4 albacore tuna steaks
- 6 tablespoons sugar, divided
- 2 tablespoons sesame seeds
- 1 green onion, sliced
- 1 clove garlic, minced
- 1 teaspoon chopped fresh ginger root
- 1/2 cup soy sauce
- 2 tablespoons sesame oil
- salt and pepper to taste

Direction

- Rub the albacore steaks with 4 tablespoons sugar. Allow to sit 30 minutes in the refrigerator.

- In a skillet over medium heat, toast the sesame seeds 5 minutes, or until lightly browned.
- In a shallow bowl, mix the remaining sugar, toasted sesame seeds, green onion, garlic, ginger, soy sauce, sesame oil, salt, and pepper.
- Put the albacore steaks in the mixture, and marinate 2 hours in the refrigerator in airtight container.
- Preheat the oven broiler.
- Throw away excess marinade and place the albacore steaks on a baking sheet. Broil to desired doneness (about 4-5 minutes per side for me) in the preheated oven.

36. Broiled Honey Lime Salmon Recipe

Serving: 4 | Prep: | Cook: 6mins | Ready in:

Ingredients

- marinade
- 2 tbsp Dijon mustard
- juice of one freshly squeezed lime
- 2 tsp olive oil
- 1 tbsp honey
- 1 1/2 tsp dried tarragon
- 2 tbsp dry sherry
- 1/4 tsp salt
- 1 1/4 lb salmon fillets 1/2 to 5/8 thick
- non stick cooking spray

Direction

- Combine marinade ingredients thoroughly.
- Place salmon fillets in shallow non-metal dish and top with Marinade turning to coat other side.
- Marinate in refrigerator for 1 hour turning once or twice.
- Preheat broiler.
- Coat broiler pan with cooking spray.
- Broil fish 4-6 inches from heating element for 5-6 minutes until fish is done (no need to turn).
- Serve with lime wedges (if desired).

37. Broiled Salmon And Miso Glaze Recipe

Serving: 4 | Prep: | Cook: 10mins | Ready in:

Ingredients

- 1 green onion, minced
- 2 tablespoons red miso
- 1 tablespoon rice vinegar
- 1 tablespoon honey
- 1 teaspoon minced fresh ginger
- 4 portions of center-cut salmon fillet
- 1 teaspoon toasted sesame seeds

Direction

- Whisk green onion, miso, vinegar, honey and ginger in a medium bowl until the honey is dissolved.
- Place salmon in a sealable plastic bag, add 3 tablespoons of the sauce and refrigerate; let marinate for 15 minutes.
- Reserve the remaining sauce.
- Preheat broiler. Line a small baking pan with foil and coat with cooking spray.
- Transfer the salmon to the pan, skinned-side down. Discard the marinade.
- Broil the salmon 4 to 6 inches from the heat source until cooked through, 6 to 10 minutes.
- Drizzle with the reserved sauce and garnish with sesame seeds.

38. Broiled Salmon With Marmalade Dijon Sauce Recipe

Serving: 4 | Prep: | Cook: 10mins | Ready in:

Ingredients

- 1/2 cup orange marmalade

- 1 tablespoon Dijon mustard
- 1/2 teaspoon garlic powder
- 1/2 teaspoon salt
- 1/4 teaspoon black pepper
- 1/8 teaspoon ground ginger
- 4 (6-ounce) salmon fillets
- cooking spray

Direction

- Preheat broiler.
- Combine first 6 ingredients in a small bowl, stirring well. Place fish on a jelly-roll pan coated with cooking spray. Brush half of marmalade mixture over fish; broil 6 minutes. Brush fish with remaining marmalade mixture; broil for 2 minutes or until fish flakes easily when tested with a fork or until desired degree of doneness.

39. Broiled Salmon With Tarragon Garlic Butter Recipe

Serving: 2 | Prep: | Cook: 10mins | Ready in:

Ingredients

- 1/4 cup butter
- 2 garlic cloves, minced
- 2 tablespoons fresh lemon juice
- 1 1/2 tbsp minced fresh tarragon or1 tsp dried, crumbled
- Freshly ground pepper to taste
- 2 (1-inch-thick) salmon fillets
- salt to taste

Direction

- Preheat broiler.
- Melt butter in small saucepan on the stove top over medium-low heat and sauté garlic for a few seconds.
- Remove from heat and add lemon juice, tarragon and pepper.
- Arrange salmon skin side down on broiler-proof pan.
- Brush with half of butter mixture.
- Season with salt.
- Broil until nearly cooked; turn over and a cook until done to personal preference.
- Transfer to plates. Reheat remaining lemon/butter sauce; spoon over salmon and serve.

40. Broiled Sour Cream And Dill Salmon Recipe

Serving: 4 | Prep: | Cook: 15mins | Ready in:

Ingredients

- 2 medium cucumbers,cut into thin slices
- 1 Tbsp. red wine vinegar
- 4 tsp. olive oil
- 1 tsp. lemon pepper seasoning
- 1/2 tsp. gradulated garlic
- 1/2 tsp. fresh dill, chopped (plus sprigs for garnish)
- 1/2 small onion, thinly sliced into rings
- 1 tsp. extra virgin olive oil
- 4 (7 oz) boneless, skin-on salmon fillets
- 1/4 cup fresh lemon juice
- 1/2 tsp. onion salt
- 1/4 cup light sour cream
- lemon slices for garnish
- salt and pepper to taste

Direction

- Using a vegetable peeler, cut cucumber into thin slices (slice up to the seed portion) and place in a small bowl.
- Add onions, vinegar, and extra virgin olive oil and mix well, season with salt and pepper to taste. Refrigerate until ready to serve.
- Place oven rack 4 to 5" from top of oven. Preheat broiler to high.
- Coat both sides of salmon fillets with olive oil.

- Place salmon, skin side up, in a shallow baking dish. Broil salmon until skin is lightly browned, about 4 to 5 minutes.
- Turn salmon over, pour lemon juice over salmon, and sprinkle with granulated garlic, onion salt and lemon pepper seasoning. Broil salmon, checking the oven often, until lightly browned, about 4 to 5 minutes.
- Combine the sour cream and dill and spread evenly over the top of each salmon fillet. Broil approximately 3 to 4 minutes or until the sour cream topping is lightly browned.
- Remove skin from fillets and serve over cucumber mixture, garnished with dill sprigs and lemon slices.

41. Broiled Tilapia With Sweet Potato Crust And Vanilla Cream Sauce Recipe

Serving: 2 | Prep: | Cook: 10mins | Ready in:

Ingredients

- 2 (6 ounce size) tilapia fillets
- ****FILLING****
- 3 sweet potatoes - cooked & peeled
- 3 teaspoons fresh lemon juice
- 4 teaspoons fresh orange juice
- 1 Tablespoon butter
- 1 teaspoon salt
- 1/2 teaspoon minced ginger
- ***CRUST***
- 3 graham crackers
- 1 cup roasted pecans
- 2 Tablespoons melted butter
- **SAUCE**
- 5 Tablespoons heavy cream
- 1 Tablespoon vanilla
- 2 Tablespoons fish stock OR water
- 1 pinch of seafood or creole seasoning

Direction

- Grind sweet potatoes, juices, butter, salt and ginger together and set aside.
- Grind the graham crackers, pecans and butter together.
- Cover the fish with the sweet potato mixture. Then sprinkle the pecan mixture over the top
- Broil the fillets until golden brown...approx. 4 minutes.
- In a small skillet, add the cream, vanilla, stock and seasoning.
- Bring to a boil and cook for a minute, until the alcohol in the vanilla is gone and the sauce coats the back of the spoon.
- Pool the sauce on a plate.
- Place the broiled fish fillet on top and serve.
- Enjoy!
- **
- -Faith, like light, should always be simple and unbending, while love like warmth, should beam forth on every side, and bend to every necessity of our brethren. - Martin Luther
- **

42. Broiled Tuna Steaks Recipe

Serving: 2 | Prep: | Cook: 16mins | Ready in:

Ingredients

- 4 tuna steaks
- 1/4 cup vegetable oil
- 1 tablespoon oregano
- 1 tablespoon basil
- 2 tablespoons lemon juice
- 2 cloves garlic
- 1 teaspoon salt

Direction

- Mix the ingredients.
- Marinade the tuna steaks at room temperature for about half an hour.
- Broil for 6-8 minutes per side.

43. Brown Sugar Glazed Salmon Recipe

Serving: 0 | Prep: | Cook: 10mins | Ready in:

Ingredients

- 2 large salmon fillets
- 2/3 cup brown sugar
- 2 Tbs honey
- 2 Tbs Dijon mustard
- 1/2 tsp salt
- chopped fresh dill to garnish

Direction

- Mix the sugar, honey, mustard and salt well. Place salmon skin side down on baking tray. Brush over the salmon.
- Broil 3 to 4 inches from heat source and broil 8 to 10 minutes or until golden glazed and done.
- Garnish with dill and lemon slices if desired
- May be served warm or room temperature
- Note: may also use salmon steaks for the recipe

44. CRISPY WEST LAKE FISH XIHU CUYU Recipe

Serving: 4 | Prep: | Cook: 20mins | Ready in:

Ingredients

- You can use either skinless or skin-on fillets here; most tasters liked the crisp texture of the cooked skin. Any thin, medium-firm white fish fillets can be substituted for the catfish, including haddock, tilapia, flounder, snapper, trout, orange roughy, tilefish, and arctic char. Keep the sauce and the fish separate until ready to serve to help preserve the crisp exterior of the fish.
- INGREDIENTS
- Sauce
- 1 tablespoon minced or grated fresh ginger
- 2 medium garlic cloves , minced or pressed through a garlic press (about 2 teaspoons)
- 1 red or green jalapeño chile , or Thai red, or serrano chile, stemmed, seeded, and chopped coarse
- 1 small Thai red, serrano, or red or green jalapeno chile , stemmed, seeded, and chopped coarse
- 3 tablespoons sugar
- 1 cup water
- 3 tablespoons red wine vinegar
- 1 tablespoon soy sauce
- 1 tablespoon Chinese rice cooking wine or dry sherry
- 1 tablespoon cornstarch
- 3 scallions , sliced thin
- fish
- 4 catfish fillets (about 6 ounces each)
- salt and ground black pepper
- 3 tablespoons cornstarch
- 1/4 cup vegetable oil
- Flipping Fish Fillets:
- To easily turn fish fillets without breaking them, use two spatulas--a regular model and an extrawide version especially designed for fish. (In the test kitchen, we use a spatula that is 8 1/2 inches wide by 3 1/4 inches deep for this job.) Using the regular spatula, gently lift the long side of the fillet. Then, supporting the fillet with the extrawide spatula, flip it so that the browned side face up.

Direction

- 1. FOR THE SAUCE: Combine the ginger, garlic, chili, and sugar together in a small heavy- bottomed saucepan and cook over medium-high heat until the sugar melts and turns golden brown, 5 to 7 minutes. Whisk the water, vinegar, soy sauce, rice wine, and cornstarch together, then carefully whisk into the saucepan – the sugar mixture will be extremely hot. Continue to simmer, stirring constantly, until the sauce is thickened, 2 to 4 minutes. Cover and set aside off the heat.

- 2. FOR THE FISH: Adjust the oven racks to the lower- and upper-middle positions, set 4 heatproof dinner plates on the racks, and heat the oven to 200 degrees. Pat the fish dry with paper towels and season both sides with salt and pepper; let stand until the fillets are glistening with moisture, about 5 minutes.
- 3. Spread the cornstarch into a wide, shallow dish. Coat both sides of the fillets with cornstarch, shake off the excess, and lay in a single layer on a baking sheet. Heat 2 tablespoons of the oil in a 12-inch non-stick skillet over high heat until shimmering. Carefully place 2 fillets in the skillet, skin side down, and immediately reduce the heat to medium-high. Cook, without moving the fish, until the edges of the fillets are opaque and the bottom is golden and crisp, about 4 1/2 minutes.
- 4. Following the illustration below, use 2 spatulas to gently flip the fillets, then continue to cook on the second side until the thickest part of the fillet easily separates into flakes when a toothpick is inserted, about 3 minutes longer. Transfer each of the fillets to a heated dinner plate in the oven. Wipe out the skillet and repeat with the remaining 2 tablespoons oil and the remaining fillets; transfer each fillet to a plate in oven. (The fish can be held in the oven for up to 10 minutes before continuing.)
- 5. Return the sauce to a brief simmer over medium-high heat. Stir in the scallions, then pour the sauce over the fish and serve immediately.

45. Caesar Baked Fish Filets Recipe

Serving: 1 | Prep: | Cook: 15mins | Ready in:

Ingredients

- 1 cod, haddock or tilapia filet
- 2 tablespoons mayonnaise
- 1 tablespoon parmesan cheese, grated
- 1 1/2 teaspoons lemon juice
- 1/4 teaspoon salt, or to taste
- dash ground black pepper
- 1/4 cup fresh breadcrumbs
- 2 tablespoons fresh parsley, minced
- lemon wedges

Direction

- Preheat oven to 450 degrees.
- Place fish filet in greased baking dish.
- Combine mayonnaise, Parmesan, lemon juice, salt and pepper.
- Spread over fish filet.
- Combine breadcrumbs and parsley.
- Sprinkle over fish.
- Bake about 10 minutes or until fish flakes easily and crumbs begin to brown.
- Serve with lemon wedges.

46. Cajun Spiced Catfish Kebabs Recipe

Serving: 4 | Prep: | Cook: 8mins | Ready in:

Ingredients

- 2 tsp. paprika
- 1 tsp. garlic powder
- 1 tsp. dried oregano
- 1 tsp. dried thyme
- 1/2 tsp. salt
- 1/2 tsp. ground red pepper
- 4 (6-ounce) catfish fillets, cut into 24 (1-inch) pieces
- 1/2 C fat-free mayonnaise
- 1 Tbl. fresh lemon juice
- 2 tsp. capers, chopped
- 2 tsp. prepared horseradish
- 2 ears corn, each cut crosswise into 8 pieces
- 3 green bell peppers, each cut into 8 wedges
- cooking spray

Direction

- Combine first 6 ingredients in a medium bowl; add catfish, tossing to coat. Cover and refrigerate 20 minutes.
- Combine mayonnaise, juice, capers, and horseradish in a small bowl; stir with a whisk. Cover and refrigerate.
- Prepare grill.
- Cook the corn in boiling water for 3 minutes, and drain.
- Thread 3 catfish pieces, 2 corn pieces, and 3 bell pepper pieces alternately onto each of 8 (12-inch) skewers.
- Place kebabs on a grill rack coated with cooking spray; grill for 4 minutes on each side or until fish flakes easily when tested with a fork.
- Serve with sauce.

47. Cant Miss Red Snapper Recipe

Serving: 4 | Prep: | Cook: 15mins | Ready in:

Ingredients

- 4 red snapper fillets, 1/2" thk - (8 oz ea)
- 1 teaspoon salt
- 1/2 teaspoon freshly-ground black pepper
- 1 cup chopped onions
- 1 green bell pepper -- chopped
- 1/2 cup butter - (1 stick)
- 1 tablespoon worcestershire sauce
- 1 cup freshly-grated Parmesan

Direction

- Season the fish with the salt and pepper. Spread the onions and pepper in a 13- by 9-inch glass baking dish and place the fish on top. Dot the fish with butter. Sprinkle with a little Worcestershire sauce.
- Bake for 12 minutes, then baste fish with pan juices. Sprinkle the fish with Parmesan and then place under the broiler for about 2 minutes or until the cheese browns.
- To serve, spoon the vegetables over the fish.

48. Caribbean Grilled Tilapia With Mango Salsa Recipe

Serving: 4 | Prep: | Cook: 20mins | Ready in:

Ingredients

- 4 fresh tilapia fillets
- 1/2 cup extra virgin olive oil
- 1/3 cup white wine
- 2 teaspoons caribbean jerk seasoning
- 1 tablespoon dried parsley flakes
- 8 ounce can sliced pineapple in its own juice
- Salsa:
- 2/3 cup chopped mango
- 2 tablespoons fresh squeezed lime juice
- 2 tablespoons fresh squeezed orange juice
- 4 rounded teaspoons jalapeno peppers very finely chopped
- 4 rounded teaspoons finely chopped red onions
- 2 rounded teaspoons finely chopped red bell pepper
- 2 rounded teaspoons finely chopped green bell pepper
- 1 teaspoon dried parsley flakes
- 1 teaspoon freshly ground black pepper

Direction

- Mix olive oil, wine and parsley then marinate fish in the mixture for 1 hour.
- Place fish on well-oiled hot grill.
- Sprinkle fish with half of the jerk seasoning and half of the pineapple juice.
- Baste some of the oil marinade on the pieces of fish.
- Place pineapple slices on grill as well.
- Turn fish over and sprinkle with remaining seasonings.
- Add pineapple juice and oil marinade as on first side.
- Flip pineapple slices.

- Serve fish with pineapple slices and top with mango salsa.
- To make salsa mix all ingredients well and refrigerate for an hour or more before serving.

49. Cashew Crusted Tilapia Recipe

Serving: 4 | Prep: | Cook: 10mins | Ready in:

Ingredients

- 1/2 C flour or Bisquick
- 1 Tbls salt
- 1 1/2 tsp pepper
- 2 large eggs
- 2 cups finely chopped cashews
- 2 9 - 10 oz tilapia fillets
- 2 Tbs butter
- 2 Tbls olive oil
- 1 lemon quartered
- chopped fresh parsly

Direction

- Using a fork, stir flour, salt and pepper in large plate to blend. Whisk eggs in a medium bowl to blend. Place Cashews on a large plate. Sprinkle fillets with salt and pepper, dredge in flour mixture, then dip in eggs to coat. Press both sides of the fillet into the nuts.
- Melt butter and oil in heavy skillet over medium heat. Add fillets to skillet and cook until coating is lightly browned and fish is cooked through - about 5 mins per side.
- Place on fillet on a plate, squeeze a little lemon on it and sprinkle some parsley and serve.

50. Catch Of The Day Weight Watchers Recipe

Serving: 4 | Prep: | Cook: 20mins | Ready in:

Ingredients

- 6 fish filets(cod, sole, flounder, halibut, tilapia, orange roughy)
- 2 eggs, lightly beaten
- 1 cup oatmeal, ground to consistency of flour
- juice of 1 or 2 lemons, to taste
- 1/2 cup white wine
- 1/2 cup chicken broth
- 2-3 T capers, to taste
- cooking spray

Direction

- Preheat large frying pan to medium-high heat for a minute or so.
- Spray well with cooking spray.
- Dip filets in oatmeal flour, then in egg, then back in oatmeal.
- Place in the pan and brown for a couple of minutes on each side.
- Once both sides are browned, squeeze lemon juice over filets.
- Add wine, chicken broth, and top with capers.
- Let simmer on low heat for approximately 15 minutes, until filets flake easily with a fork.

51. Catfish Fillets With Egyptian Tahini Sauce Recipe

Serving: 2 | Prep: | Cook: 10mins | Ready in:

Ingredients

- 1 garlic clove
- 1/4 cup well-stirred tahini
- 1/3 cup water
- 1 1/2 tablespoons fresh lemon juice
- 1/4 teaspoon ground cumin
- 1/4 teaspoon salt
- 2 teaspoons coriander seeds
- two 6-ounce catfish fillets
- 1 tablespoon olive oil
- 2 tablespoons coarsely chopped fresh flat-leafed parsley leaves

Direction

- Coarsely chop garlic and in a blender purée with tahini, water, lemon juice, cumin, and salt until smooth.
- Using the flat side of a large knife coarsely crush coriander seeds. Pat catfish dry and season with salt and pepper. In a 10-inch non-stick skillet heat oil over moderately high heat until hot but not smoking and sauté fish 2 minutes. Turn fish over, sprinkling crushed coriander around it, and sauté 2 minutes more, or until just cooked through. Divide tahini sauce between 2 plates and top with fish, crushed coriander and oil from skillet, and parsley.

52. Catfish Tacos With Thai Cabbage Slaw Recipe

Serving: 6 | Prep: | Cook: 25mins | Ready in:

Ingredients

- Tacos: -----------
- 2 pounds catfish fillets (about 3 fillets)
- 1 package of flour tortillas
- 1 avocados, skinned, pitted, and thinly sliced
- 1 handful fresh cilantro leaves, rough chopped or hand shredded
- 1 limes cut into wedges
- oil for the grill
- For the Thai Slaw Dressing: -----------
- 1 Tbsp fish sauce
- 1/4 cup freshly squeezed lime juice (from about 2 juicy limes)
- 2 tsp sesame oil
- 1 tsp red chili paste
- 1/2 cup coconut milk, more if needed
- 1/2 cup peanut butter
- 1 tsp honey, or to taste
- red pepper flakes (optional and to taste)
- For the Thai Slaw: ------------
- 2 cups thinly sliced red cabbage (about 1/4 to 1/2 of a small cabbage)
- 2 carrots, shredded
- 1 daikon radish, shredded
- 1/2 medium red onion, thinly sliced

Direction

- Thai Slaw Dressing: ------------
- Whisk fish sauce, lime juice, sesame oil, chili paste, coconut milk and peanut butter together in small pot over medium-low heat.
- Cook, stirring often, for 5 minutes.
- Thin with coconut milk if needed to obtain a sauce that pours easily.
- Taste and adjust seasoning with honey and red pepper flakes.
- Thai Slaw: ------------
- Combine red cabbage, carrots, daikon and red onion in a large bowl.
- Toss with half of the slaw dressing.
- Set remaining dressing aside for serving with the tacos.
- Catfish Tacos: ------------
- Preheat grill to medium heat.
- Rub both sides of fish with a little oil.
- When grill is hot, use tongs to rub the grate with an oiled paper towel.
- Grill fish 5 to 7 minutes on each side or until fish is opaque and flakes easily with a fork.
- Meanwhile, wrap a stack of tortillas in foil and place on grill over low heat, turning once while the fish cooks.
- When the fish is done, remove it from the grill and cut into pieces.
- Pile fish in warm tortillas. Top with Thai slaw, sliced avocado, cilantro leaves and extra Thai slaw dressing.
- Serve with lime wedges.

53. Catfish And Okra With Pecan Butter Sauce Recipe

Serving: 4 | Prep: | Cook: 30mins | Ready in:

Ingredients

- 1 (10-oz) package frozen whole baby okra, thawed and rinsed
- 12 oz grape tomatoes (2 cups)
- 2 tablespoons vegetable oil
- 1/2 teaspoon salt
- 1/4 teaspoon black pepper
- 4 (1/2-lb) catfish fillets
- 2 teaspoons Old Bay Seasoning
- 1 (10-oz) package frozen corn, thawed
- 3/4 stick (6 tablespoons) unsalted butter
- 1/2 cup pecans (2 oz), coarsely chopped
- 1 teaspoon fresh lemon juice
- Garnish: lemon wedges

Direction

- Put oven racks in upper and lower thirds of oven and preheat oven to 500°F.
- Toss okra and tomatoes with oil, salt, and pepper in a bowl. Spread in a large shallow baking pan and roast in lower third of oven until tomato skins begin to burst, about 10 minutes.
- Meanwhile, pat fillets dry and arrange in another large shallow baking pan. Sprinkle both sides with 1 1/2 teaspoons (total) Old Bay seasoning.
- When tomato skins begin to burst, add corn to vegetables in lower third of oven and put fish in upper third of oven. Roast fish and vegetables until fish is just cooked through, about 10 minutes.
- While fish roasts, melt butter in a 10-inch heavy skillet over moderate heat, then add pecans and remaining 1/2 teaspoon Old Bay seasoning. Cook, stirring occasionally, until nuts are golden and butter is deep golden, about 3 minutes. Remove from heat and stir in lemon juice. Serve fish over vegetables and top with sauce.

54. Cedar Plank Halibut Tacos With Chipotle Avocado Cream Recipe

Serving: 4 | Prep: | Cook: 20mins | Ready in:

Ingredients

- For Halibut:
- 4 pieces fresh wild halibut filets, 6 to 8 ounces each
- 1 teaspoon finely grated lime peel
- smoked paprika, kosher salt and freshly ground black pepper
- olive oil, for drizzling
- For avocado Chipotle Cream:
- 1/2 cup mayonnaise
- 1/2 cup sour cream
- 1 small ripe avocado, cubed
- 1 small garlic clove
- 1 chipotle pepper in adobo (or use chipotle powder to taste)
- 2 tablespoons fresh lime juice
- Pinch of salt
- Serve with:
- fresh corn tortillas, finely shredded napa cabbage, lime wedges

Direction

- Soak cedar plank for at least 30 minutes in water. Season halibut with smoked paprika, kosher salt and freshly ground black pepper. Drizzle lightly with olive oil.
- Heat a charcoal grill. Place halibut on dried off cedar plank and grill until fish is cooked, about 16-20 minutes.
- Take plank off grill, tent fish lightly with foil and allow resting for 10-15 minutes.
- For Avocado Chipotle Cream, place all ingredients in food processor and pulse until smooth. Transfer to small serving bowl.
- Gently flake fish into large chucks and put on serving platter. Serve with warm corn tortillas, avocado chipotle cream, shredded cabbage and limes wedges. Garnish with cilantro, optional.

55. Cedar Plank Salmon Recipe

Serving: 4 | Prep: | Cook: 15mins | Ready in:

Ingredients

- 2 tbsp grainy mustard
- 2 tbsp ketchup
- 1 tbsp chopped fresh rosemary
- 2 tbsp olive oil
- 1/2 tsp chili powder
- salt and freshly ground pepper
- One 2 lb piece of raw salmon

Direction

- Combine mustard, ketchup, rosemary, olive oil, chili powder, salt and pepper.
- Spread over salmon and marinate for 30 minutes.
- Heat grill to high heat.
- Place soaked cedar plank on grill and leave for 3 to 4 minutes or until you can smell or see smoke.
- Immediately turn plank, salt it liberally and place fish on top, skin-side down.
- Close cover and cook for 12 to15 minutes or until fish is just cooked.
- Remove plank from grill and slip salmon off, onto serving platter.

56. Cedar Plank Salmon With Orange Balsamic Glaze Recipe

Serving: 4 | Prep: | Cook: 20mins | Ready in:

Ingredients

- 1/2 cup freshly squeezed orange juice
- zest of 1 orange
- 1/4 cup sugar
- 1/4 cup balsamic vinegar
- 1 tablespoon extra-virgin olive oil
- 2 cloves garlic, finely chopped
- 1 tablespoon finely chopped fresh rosemary
- kosher salt & freshly ground black pepper to taste
- 4 salmon steaks or filets (about 6 ounces each)

Direction

- Place orange juice, zest and sugar in a saucepan over high heat and bring to boil. Reduce by half and cool.
- Place reduction along with the rest of the ingredients in a large sealable plastic bag. Shake well. Add salmon and refrigerate 1 hour. Meanwhile, soak a cedar plank for 1 hour and preheat charcoal grill.
- Remove steaks/filets from marinade. Position salmon on soaked cedar plank and place over hottest part of your grill. Close lid and grill until salmon to 120 degrees internal. Remove from grill, cover with foil and rest for 5 minutes.
- Note: while the salmon is grilling, we like to throw down fresh corn on the cob that has been rubbed with olive oil and sprinkled with kosher salt. The corn picks up the wonderful flavor from the cedar. After it's nicely caramelized, take the cobs off the grill and rub butter all over them... enjoy!

57. Ceviche Recipe

Serving: 10 | Prep: | Cook: 5mins | Ready in:

Ingredients

- 3 LBS TILAPIA
- 1/2 LB PRE-COOKEDSHRIMP
- 2 MED. onions
- 5-7 tomatoes
- 1-2 BUNCHES cilantro
- 6-8 limes
- 3-4 TABLESPOONS salt

- 1 BOTTLE VALENTINAS hot sauce (OR WHAT YOU PREFER)
- 1 PKG TOSTADAS

Direction

- 1. The traditional way to cook the ceviche is to soak the Tilapia in the lime. To speed this up, bring a small pan of water to a boil (just enough to cover the Tilapia). Once boiling, lay the Tilapia in the pan about 3-5 minutes; the fish will turn white and start to fall apart. Drain all the water, press all the water out of the fish. Don't leave any water.
- Place fish in bowl and with a fork, shred it to pieces. Add the shrimp into the bowl.
- Dice the onion & tomato. Place them in the bowl and also shrimp. Cut cilantro into very small pieces, add that to the bowl. Mix all ingredients in bowl together.
- Cut the limes in half start with about 6 (you can always add more to your taste). Take the lime and squeeze all of them into the bowl, mix together. Then sprinkle 3 tbsp salt over the bowl. If it seems dry, continue to add lime.
- Then place in fridge covered for about 2 hrs. (The longer you let it sit the more flavor).
- Then serve in bowls with hot sauce and tostadas. You may need to add more salt at this time. Enjoy!!

58. Cheesy Flounder Fillets Recipe

Serving: 4 | Prep: | Cook: 20mins | Ready in:

Ingredients

- 1/3 cup light mayonnaise
- 1/3 cup cheddar cheese, shredded
- 4 flounder fillets, 6-ounces each
- 1 package (6.1 ounces) tomato lentil couscous mix
- 1 box (10-ounces) frozen spinach

Direction

- Preheat oven at 400F.
- Spray a baking dish with nonstick cooking spray.
- Mix together the mayo and cheddar cheese. Place the fillets in the dish and fold in half. Evenly divide the mayo mixture over each and spread evenly.
- Bake fillets for 20 minutes or until fish flakes easily.
- While fish is baking, prepare couscous and spinach following package directions.
- Serve fillets with couscous and spinach alongside.

59. Chilled Poached Haddock With Cucumber Relish Recipe

Serving: 4 | Prep: | Cook: 65mins | Ready in:

Ingredients

- relish
- 2 cucumbers, peeled, seeded and finely diced
- 2 T red onion, finely diced
- 2 T mint, finely chopped
- ½ jalapeno pepper, seeded and finely diced
- 1 C finely diced watermelon
- 1 T sugar
- 2 T fresh lime juice
- 1 ½ tsp rice wine vinegar
- ¼ tsp salt
- haddock
- 1 C water
- ½ C white wine
- 1 small onion, sliced thin
- 12 sprigs parsley, divided
- ¼ tsp salt
- 1 ½ lbs fresh haddock fillets
- lemon wedges for garnish

Direction

- Relish

- Combine all ingredients in a glass or ceramic bowl, mix well and chill
- Haddock
- In a large saucepan with a tight fitting lid. Place water, wine, onion, 4 sprigs of parsley and salt
- Bring to a boil over high heat, then lower heat to medium and simmer
- Add fish fillets, skin side up
- Poach 5 minutes, uncovered
- Remove pan from heat, cover and let sit another 5 minutes
- Check to see if fish is cooked, if not replace lid and let sit another 5 minutes
- When fish is done, remove lid
- When fish is cool enough to handle, slip a sharp knife under skin and remove
- Carefully remove fish to a serving platter and cool 20 minutes at room temp
- Cover loosely with plastic wrap and refrigerate at least an hour
- When ready to serve, arrange remaining parsley sprigs around fish, along with lemon wedges
- Serve haddock chilled with cucumber relish on the side

60. Citrus Red Miso Ginger Glazed Halibut Recipe

Serving: 4 | Prep: | Cook: 15mins | Ready in:

Ingredients

- 4 halibut filets approx. 2 inches in thickness or any firm white fish
- flour for coating
- salt and pepper to taste
- 1 tsp of olive oil
- 1 clove of garlic, minced
- 1 tbsp of fresh ginger, grated
- 1/3 c orange juice
- 1 tbsp sugar
- 2 stalks of green onion, chopped
- 1/4 c of red miso (Akamiso)

Direction

- Lightly salt and pepper halibuts.
- Coat lightly with flour.
- Heat oil in pan and add halibut filets. Cook over medium at 2 minutes per side. Turn only once.
- Shake pan slightly to avoid sticking.
- Remove and place in foil pan skin side up. Finish cooking in a 350 degrees oven for another 5 to 7 minutes. Check occasionally.
- Add ginger and garlic to pan. Slowly add orange juice and scrap some of the drippings from the pan.
- Add red miso and whisk lightly. Add sugar to dissolve and salt and pepper to taste.
- Once sauce thickens, add the green onion.
- Serve on top of fish with rice and salad.

61. Citrus Salmon Recipe

Serving: 2 | Prep: | Cook: 12mins | Ready in:

Ingredients

- 2 ea 8 oz. salmon fillets
- 1 lemon, zested and segmented
- 1 orange, zested and segmented
- ½ cup orange juice
- ¼ cup lemon juice
- 1 jalapeño pepper
- 2 tablespoons fresh cilantro, chopped
- 2 sprigs fresh cilantro for garnish
- 2 tablespoons olive oil or vegetable oil

Direction

- Remove skin from salmon fillets; discard.
- Slice 8-10 very thin rounds from the tip of the jalapeño; set aside. Cut remaining pepper in half, remove and discard seeds, then mince.
- Mince lemon and orange zest, then combine in a 1-quart-size Ziploc storage bag with lemon

juice, orange juice, jalapeño and cilantro; add salmon fillets, close bag, and set on a plate – marinate in refrigerator for 30 minutes.

- While salmon marinates, heat oven to 400°F and segment lemon and orange.
- To segment, cut top and bottom off of lemon and orange; stand upright. Using a very sharp knife, run the blade down from top to bottom, removing the white pith. Turn and continue until all pith has been removed. Lay citrus on its side; use blade to cut segments of flesh from between the white membrane; reserve.
- After salmon has marinated, heat 2 tablespoons olive oil in an oven-safe skillet over medium heat. Remove salmon from Ziploc, shake loose excess marinade, and carefully lay each fillet in pan (be careful – oil will pop and sizzle). Cook for 2 minutes, then turn each fillet over; top each with even amounts of lemon and orange segments, then transfer skillet to oven to finish cooking (about 8-10 minutes).
- Remove from oven; use spatula to lift each fillet from pan; place on a plate. Garnish with a fresh sprig of cilantro and thin-shaved pieces of jalapeño. Serve while hot!

62. Citrus Salmon With Orange Relish Recipe

Serving: 4 | Prep: | Cook: 15mins | Ready in:

Ingredients

- Citrus Salmon:
- 1/4 cup orange juice
- 2 Tbs. olive oil
- 1 1/2 tps. thyme leaves, divided
- 4 salmon fillets (about 1 pound)
- 1 Tbs. brown sugar
- 1 tps. paprika
- 1/2 tps. salt
- orange Relish:
- 1/2 tps. grated orange peel
- 2 seedless oranges, pelled, sectioned and cut into 1/2 -inch pieces
- 2 Tbs. chopped red bell pepper
- 1 Tbs. honey
- 1 Tbs. chopped red onion
- 1 Tbs. chopped fresh parsley
- 1/2 tps. ground ginger

Direction

- For the Salmon, mix orange juice, oil and 1 tsp. of the thyme in a small bowl. Place salmon in a large resealable plastic bag or glass dish. Add marinade; turn to coat well. Refrigerate 30 minutes or longer for extra flavor. For the Relish, mix all ingredients in medium bowl. Cover. Refrigerate until ready to serve.
- Preheat oven to 400F. Mix brown sugar, paprika, remaining 1/2 tsp. thyme and salt in small bowl. Remove salmon from marinade. Discard any remaining marinade> Rub salmon evenly with paprika mixture. Place salmon on foil-lined baking pan.
- Bake 10 to 15 minutes or until fish flakes easily. Serve salmon with the relish.
- Recipe McCormick & Co ENJOY

63. Classic Baked Catfish Recipe

Serving: 6 | Prep: | Cook: 20mins | Ready in:

Ingredients

- Skinned catfish fillets
- Squeeze butter
- lemon juice
- Donnie's cajun seasoning Mix (or equivalent ingredients) (Recipe on my recipe page)
- onion powder
- dried parsley
- Italian bread crumbs
- paprika

Direction

- Wash and dry catfish fillets.
- Preheat oven to 375 deg.
- Grease a glass (Pyrex) 13x8x2 inch baking dish with butter. (A lot, so that you end up with it being ¼ inch thick after it melts)
- Put dish into oven until the butter melts. Then remove from oven.
- Arrange fillets in the dish then flip over so that both sides are covered heavy in butter. (Make sure that the skin sides of the fillets are facing down when finished)
- Sprinkle seasoning mix, onion powder and dried parsley over fillets.
- Drizzle with plenty of lemon juice.
- Distribute a light coating of Italian bread crumbs evenly over fillets.
- Top with a good sprinkling of paprika for color.
- Put into oven at 375 deg. and bake for 20 minutes or until fish is done.
- If browning is desired, place under broiler for 2 to 3 minutes.

64. Classic Poached Salmon Recipe

Serving: 10 | Prep: | Cook: 20mins | Ready in:

Ingredients

- Two 2 lb center-cut salmon pieces, bones removed, skin on
- salt and freshly ground pepper
- 12 cups Court Bouillon (recipe follows)
- ============================
- Garnish
- seedless cucumber
- lemon slices
- watercress
- ============================
- Court Bouillon
- Use this for salmon or other large fish.
- Court Bouillon can be strained after using, refrigerated or frozen up to six months.
- Add water to top it up.
- 12 cups water
- 1 cup dry white wine
- 1/2 cup wine vinegar
- 2 onions, sliced
- 2 carrots, sliced
- 2 bay leaves
- 6 stalks parsley
- 1 tsp dried thyme
- 1 tbsp whole peppercorns

Direction

- Preheat oven to 450°F
- Season each piece of salmon with salt and pepper, and place one on top of the other.
- Measure salmon horizontally at its thickest part.
- Wrap salmon in cheesecloth and place in buttered baking dish.
- Bring court bouillon to boil and pour over fish. It should come three-quarters of the way up the fish.
- Cover dish with foil and place on baking sheet.
- Transfer to oven and cook for 5 minutes per inch.
- Remove from oven, uncover and cool in broth.
- Place on serving platter, using the cheesecloth to help with the transfer.
- Undo cheesecloth and remove top layer of skin.
- Using cheesecloth again, turn salmon over and place skinned side down on serving platter.
- Remove the cheesecloth and top layer of skin.
- Thinly slice cucumber on a mandolin or slicer.
- Bring a pot of water to a boil, immerse cucumber slices and bring back to boil.
- Immediately drain.
- Pat cucumber slices dry.
- Overlap on top of fish to simulate scales.
- Decorate platter with lemon slices and watercress.
- Slice and serve with Green Herb Mayonnaise.
- ============================
- Court Bouillon
- In a large pot on high heat, bring all the ingredients to a boil.

- Reduce heat and simmer for 15 minutes.

65. Coconut Crusted Red Snapper Recipe

Serving: 4 | Prep: | Cook: 15mins | Ready in:

Ingredients

- Four 8 oz. red snapper fillets with skin (boned, rinsed, and patted dry)
- 1/2 cup shredded coconut (unsweetened)
- 1/2 cup flour
- 2 teaspoons curry powder
- 1 teaspoon ground coriander
- 1 teaspoon ground cumin
- 1 teaspoon black pepper
- 1 teaspoon salt
- 1 egg
- 1/2 cup milk
- 1 Tablespoon olive oil

Direction

- In a shallow bowl combine coconut, 1/4 cup flour, curry powder, coriander, cumin, black pepper, and salt.
- Mix the ingredients together until evenly combined.
- In another shallow bowl whisk together the egg and the milk.
- Place the remaining 1/4 cup flour in a shallow bowl.
- For each fillet: working with the skin side only, press each fillet into the flour, then into the egg/milk mixture, and then into the coconut mixture.
- Heat the 1 Tablespoon of olive oil in a large sauté pan until hot. Then add the fillets to the pan, coconut side down.
- Cook 3 minutes. Then turn and cook until done, about one minute more.

66. Cod And Potato Fritters Recipe

Serving: 6 | Prep: | Cook: 10mins | Ready in:

Ingredients

- 1/2 pound desalted cod flakes (if using fresh, lightly fry and chop)
- 2 medium boiled potatoes, mashed (better if steamed or microwaved, so they do not absorb so much water)
- 1/2 onion, finely chopped
- 2 beaten eggs
- 2 garlic cloves, finely chopped
- 1/4 cup fresh parsley, finely chopped
- 1/4 cup beer (any kind is OK)
- 1 tsp baking powder
- 3 Tbsp all purpose flour
- 2 cups of extra virgin spanish olive oil

Direction

- In a medium bowl place cod, potatoes, onion, eggs, garlic and parsley. Mix well.
- Add beer, baking powder and flour, 2 Tbsp. first and if the mix is too light to handle it, then add the other Tbsp. Mixture should be very similar to muffin dough, thick and able to maintain its shape when rounded with a tablespoon.
- Let it rest for at least 1/2 hour so the fritters become tastier, fluffy and lighter when fried.
- Heat the olive oil in a deep pan as fritters should be able to "swim" in the oil.
- When oil is hot but not smoking, pour the mixture by heaping tablespoons into the pan and let it fry for about 2 minutes on each side until golden and puffy.
- Drain on paper towel and serve immediately.
- They are delicious served with a side bowl of garlic mayonnaise.
- NOTE: you can keep and reuse the oil as it will not become "dirty" after these fritters.

67. Cod In Charmoula Sauce Recipe

Serving: 6 | Prep: | Cook: 60mins | Ready in:

Ingredients

- fish and Vegetables:
- 1 pound medium red boiling potatoes
- 2 tablespoons olive oil
- 2 green or yellow bell peppers, cut into 1/4-inch-wide strips
- 2 medium tomatoes, cut crosswise into 1/4-inch-thick slices
- 3 pounds haddock or cod fillets, skinned and cut into 6 pieces
- 2 tablespoons fresh lemon juice
- Charmoula Sauce:
- 1/2 cup coarsely chopped fresh cilantro leaves
- 1/2 cup coarsely chopped fresh flat-leaf parsley
- 5 garlic cloves, coarsely chopped
- 1/3 cup fresh lemon juice
- 2 teaspoons sweet paprika
- 2 teaspoons salt
- 1 1/2 teaspoons ground cumin
- 1/4 teaspoon cayenne
- 1/2 cup olive oil

Direction

- To make the fish and vegetables:
- Preheat oven to 425 degrees F. Prick each potato once with a fork, then rub potatoes with 1/2 tablespoon oil. Roast on a baking sheet in middle of oven until just tender, about 25 minutes. Cool to room temperature and cut crosswise into 1/4-inch-thick slices. Leave oven on.
- Heat remaining 1 1/2 tablespoons oil in a 12-inch heavy skillet over moderately high heat until hot but not smoking, then sauté bell peppers, stirring, until just tender, 6 to 8 minutes.
- Spread potato slices evenly in an oiled 13 by 9 by 2-inch glass baking dish and season with salt and pepper. Top with peppers, then tomatoes and fish, seasoning each layer with salt and pepper. Sprinkle fish with lemon juice.
- To make the Chermoula Sauce:
- Puree all sauce ingredients except oil in a food processor or blender. With motor running, add oil in a slow stream. Pour sauce evenly over fish and bake in middle of oven until fish is just cooked through, 25 to 30 minutes.

68. Cod In Coconut Tomato Sauce Recipe

Serving: 4 | Prep: | Cook: 25mins | Ready in:

Ingredients

- 3 tbsp. vegetable or olive oil
- 4 cod fillets (or steaks), can use any other firm fish
- salt and pepper to taste
- 1 large onion, chopped
- 4 garlic cloves, minced
- 1 red bell pepper, seeded and chopped
- 1 tsp. ground coriander
- 1 tsp. ground cumin
- 1 tsp. ground turmeric
- 1 tsp. garam masala
- 1 (14 oz. can) chopped fire-roasted tomatoes, or other canned tomatoes
- 1 cup coconut milk
- 2 tbsp. chopped fresh cilantro, or parsely

Direction

- Heat the oil in a non-stick skillet. Season the fish with salt and pepper and add to the skillet. Fry until browned on both sides, but not cooked all the way through. Remove to the plate.
- Add the onion, garlic, red bell pepper to the skillet. Sautee for about 5 minutes, or until soft. Add the spices and cook for another minute.
- Add the tomatoes and coconut milk, bring to the boil, reduce the heat and simmer for about

8 minutes, or until the liquid is mostly reduced and the sauce is thickened.

- Add the fish to the pan, cover with sauce and simmer gently for another 5 minutes, or until cooked all the way.
- Stir in cilantro or parsley.
- Serve immediately over rice, spoon the sauce over the fish.

69. Cod Veracruz Recipe

Serving: 4 | Prep: | Cook: 20mins | Ready in:

Ingredients

- 1 lb. fresh or thawed frozen cod OR haddock fillets
- 1 can (10 3/4 oz.) Campbell's® condensed tomato soup (Regular or 25% Less Sodium)
- 1 can (10 1/2 oz.) Campbell's® condensed chicken broth
- 1/3 cup Pace® Thick & chunky salsa OR Pace® Picante Sauce
- 1 tbsp. lime juice
- 2 tsp. chopped fresh cilantro
- 1 tsp. dried oregano leaves, crushed
- 1/4 tsp. garlic powder OR 1 clove garlic, minced
- 4 cups hot cooked rice

Direction

- Place fish in 2-qt. shallow baking dish.
- Mix soup, broth, salsa, lime juice, cilantro, oregano and garlic powder. Pour over fish.
- Bake at 400°F. for 20 min. or until fish is done.

70. Cod With Italian Crumb Topping Recipe

Serving: 4 | Prep: | Cook: 12mins | Ready in:

Ingredients

- 1/4 C fine dry bread Crumbs
- 2 Tbs. grated parmesan cheese
- 1 Tbs. cornmeal
- 1 tsp. olive oil
- 1/2 tsp. italian seasoning
- 1/8 tsp. garlic powder
- 1/8 tsp. ground black pepper
- 2 Tbs. light mayonnaise
- 1 tsp. fresh lemon juice
- 4 (3 ounce) cod Fillets

Direction

- Preheat oven to 450 degrees.
- In a small shallow bowl, stir together the bread crumbs, Parmesan cheese, cornmeal, olive oil, Italian seasoning, garlic powder and pepper; set aside.
- Mix together mayonnaise and lemon juice; set aside.
- Coat the rack of a broiling pan with cooking spray.
- Place the cod on the rack, folding under any thin edges of the filets.
- Brush each piece of filet with the mayonnaise mixture, then spoon the crumb mixture evenly on top.
- Bake for 10 to 12 minutes, or until the fish flakes easily when tested with a fork and is opaque all the way through.

71. Cod With Leeks And Potatoes Recipe

Serving: 4 | Prep: | Cook: 40mins | Ready in:

Ingredients

- 5 shallots, peeled and finely diced
- ½ cup dry red wine
- ½ cup red wine vinegar
- 3 garlic cloves, peeled

- ½ lb leeks (white part only), cut into a medium dice
- ½ lb potatoes, peeled and cut into small dice
- ½ cup white wine
- 1 cup fish stock
- 4 cod fillets, about 7 ounces each
- 3 ounces unsalted butter
- ½ cup grape seed or vegetable oil
- 3 Tbsp chopped chives
- 2 ounces red cabbage, julienned very thin

Direction

- Put the shallots, red wine, and red wine vinegar in a non-reactive pot and simmer gently for about 15 minutes, until the shallots are very tender and the liquid has reduced considerably. It should get thick, but don't let it dry out and start to burn.
- Blanch the garlic three times, three minutes each time, changing the water after each blanching. Place the blanched garlic in cold water, and when cool, slice garlic lengthwise into strips.
- Season the leeks and potatoes with salt and freshly ground black pepper, and sweat them in an ounce of butter over medium heat for about three minutes.
- Add the white wine to the leeks and potatoes and continue simmering for about 5 more minutes, until the wine reduces and the vegetables (especially the potatoes) start to soften.
- Add the fish stock to the leeks and potatoes and simmer for 5 more minutes.
- Season the cod fillets with salt and pepper. Heat a sauté pan over medium high heat. Add one ounce of oil.
- Add ½ ounce of butter and place the fish fillets in the pan, skin side up. Cook until the fillets are brown on one side, then turn them over and cook just until done. Be careful not to overcook them.
- In another sauté pan, heat the remaining oil and sauté the garlic slices until they are light brown. Be very careful not to burn them.
- Add the remaining ounce of butter to the leeks and potatoes and whisk until the butter is melted. Continue stirring for a minute or two, then place the warm, thick potato/leek mixture on four soup plates. Lay a fish fillet on top.
- Add ½ ounce of butter to the reduction of shallots, wine, and wine vinegar and melt over low heat, stirring constantly. Add 1 Tbsp. chopped chives. Put one Tbsp. of this mixture on top of each fish filler. Sprinkle with the remaining chopped chives, a bit of the julienned cabbage and a few slices of the sautéed garlic.
- Note: When you sauté the fish fillets, make sure your pan is actually hot enough -- if you dump the fillets into a pan that is just warm, your fillets are going to take forever to cook and they're going to come out gummy. Not the effect you're looking for. Fish stock should be relatively easy to find (probably frozen) in any quality grocery or specialty food store. You can always make your own -- there are plenty of online recipes.

72. Cod With Fried Capers Recipe

Serving: 4 | Prep: | Cook: 20mins | Ready in:

Ingredients

- 4 cod steaks
- 1/2 teaspoon salt
- 1 teaspoon freshly ground black pepper
- 2 tablespoons grated lemon peel
- 3 tablespoons minced chives
- 5 tablespoons butter
- vegetable oil
- 2 tablespoons capers

Direction

- Preheat oven to 350.
- Pat fish dry with paper towels then sprinkle with salt and pepper and place in baking dish.

- Sprinkle with lemon peel and chives and dot with butter.
- Bake 12 minutes.
- While the fish bakes put 1/2" oil in a small saucepan set over high heat.
- Pat capers dry with paper towels.
- Add capers to hot oil and cook 2 minutes.
- Immediately remove with a slotted spoon to paper towels.
- Place fish on warm plates then divide the cooking juices among them and sprinkle with capers. Serve at once.

73. Cod With Tomatoes And Onions Recipe

Serving: 4 | Prep: | Cook: 15mins | Ready in:

Ingredients

- 1 Tbsp olive oil
- 1 small red chilli, finely chopped
- 4 cloves garlic, chopped
- 2 onions, chopped
- 1 19 oz can cherry tomatoes
- 1 10 oz can diced tomatoes (or use one 28 oz can diced tomatoes if you don't have cherry tomatoes
- 1 tsp thyme
- salt and pepper to taste
- 4 cod fillets, skin removed

Direction

- Heat oil in large skillet
- Add chilli, garlic, and onions.
- Sauté for 3 minutes or until beginning to soften
- Add other ingredients except fish
- Bring to a boil and simmer for 7 minutes
- Add fish and cover with sauce
- Cover skillet and cook for about 7 more minutes, or until fish is cooked through.

74. Copycat Red Lobster Trout Vera Cruz Recipe

Serving: 2 | Prep: | Cook: 25mins | Ready in:

Ingredients

- 4 trout fillets
- butter
- salt and pepper
- -------------------------
- --Marinade:
- 1/4 cup black olives, sliced
- 1/4 cup green olives, sliced
- 1/2 cup olive oil
- 1/2 cup white wine
- 1 tsp oregano
- 1/2 cup onions, chopped
- 1/2 cup green bell peppers, chopped
- 1/2 cup tomatoes, chopped

Direction

- Mix marinade and let sit 5 minutes.
- Brush fish with butter, and sprinkle with salt and pepper and place in a baking dish.
- Pour marinade over the fish and bake at 350° for 20-25 minutes.

75. Cornbread Coated Catfish With Cucumber Sauce Recipe

Serving: 4 | Prep: | Cook: 255mins | Ready in:

Ingredients

- 1 cup chopped, seeded cucumber
- 1 cup plain fat-free yogurt
- 1/4 cup diced red pepper
- 2 Tbsp. chopped fresh parsley
- 1 1/2 Tbsp. prepared horseradish
- 1/4 tsp. salt
- 1/2 cup bottled Italian salad dressing

- 2 eggs, slightly beaten
- 2 1/2 cups cornbread stuffing mix
- 1 1/2 lb. catfish fillets

Direction

- For cucumber sauce, in a small bowl combine first 6 ingredients, blend well. Cover and chill at least 15 minutes before serving. May be several hours ahead.
- In shallow dish, combine salad dressing and egg, blend well, Process cornbread stuffing mix in food processor until finely ground, place in second shallow dish. Coat fish fillets evenly in dressing and egg mixture and then in cornbread crumbs. Place on waxed paper lined platter, cover and chill up to 4 hours.
- Preheat oven to 400F. Arrange catfish on greased baking sheet. Bake for 12 minutes or until fish flakes with a fork.
- Serve with cucumber sauce, lemon slices and your favorite fish sides.

76. Creamed Salmon And Asparagus On Garlic Toast Recipe

Serving: 2 | Prep: | Cook: 20mins | Ready in:

Ingredients

- 3 to 6 oz. cooked salmon (or a 3 to 4 oz can)
- 5 tbsp butter, separated (2,1,2)
- I clove garlic, minced
- 1 tbsp olive oil
- 1/2 lb asparagus, trimmed and cut into 1" pieces
- 1 small shallot, chopped
- 2 tbsp flour
- 1 1/2 cup milk
- 1 tbsp Dijon mustard (nice spicy one! I used a horseradish dijon)
- 3/4 tsp dried dill (or 1 tbsp chopped fresh)
- salt and pepper to taste
- 2 thick slices Italian bread
- 2 tbsp chopped fresh parsley or fresh dill

Direction

- Place 2 tbsp. butter in a small saucepan or microwave safe bowl with the garlic. Melt butter and set aside.
- In skillet, melt another 1 tbsp. of butter with 1 tbsp. olive oil. Add chopped shallot and cook for 2 or 3 minutes. Add asparagus and cook until asparagus is tender, but still bright green. Remove asparagus with slotted spoon and set aside. Add remaining 2 tbsp. butter to skillet. When melted, whisk in flour to create a roux. Whisk in milk slowly, and bring to a boil, stirring often. Add mustard, dill, flaked salmon and asparagus, and heat through.
- Meanwhile, brush bread with butter-garlic mixture and toast in toaster oven, under broiler or on a grill pan/griddle until golden.
- Place a slice of bread on each plate, top with some of the asparagus and spoon creamed salmon mixture over top. Garnish with chopped parsley or dill.

77. Creamy Salmon Pockets Recipe

Serving: 4 | Prep: | Cook: 20mins | Ready in:

Ingredients

- 4 fresh salmon steaks
- 4 Tbsp light cream
- 1 tsp fresh dill
- white pepper and salt to taste

Direction

- Rinse salmon steaks under cold running water. Pat dry and season with dill, pepper and salt.
- Prepare 4 aluminum foil, each big enough to largely hold one piece of fish.

- Arrange seasoned fish in the middle of the aluminum foil and pour 1 Tbsp. of cream on top of each steak.
- Loosely close foil over the fish, forming pockets.
- Place pockets on a baking sheet and bake in preheated 375°F oven for about 20 minutes, until fish flakes easily with a fork.

78. Crispy Crusted Flounder Recipe

Serving: 4 | Prep: | Cook: 20mins | Ready in:

Ingredients

- 1 cup tomato, seeded, chopped
- 1 cup leeks, thinly sliced
- 1/2 cup green bell pepper, chopped
- 1 Tbs. garlic minced
- 4 flounder fillets (6 oz.each)
- 1/2 cup coarse bread crumbs
- 1/2 cup parmesan cheese, grated
- 1/2 cup plain potato chips, crushed
- 1/2 tps. paprika
- 1/4 tps. cayenne
- 2 Tbs. butter, melted
- 1 Tbs. scallion, thinly sliced
- lemon wedges

Direction

- Preheat oven to 450 F.
- Combine first four ingredients in a bowl. Spread on a baking sheet coated with cooking spray. Arrange fillets on top of vegetables; season with salt and pepper to taste.
- Combine crumbs and next four ingredients; toss with melted butter. Divide crumb mixture evenly over each fillet, pressing into the fish. Bake 20 minutes or until fillets flake easily when tested with a fork.
- Sprinkle with scallion and serve with lemon wedges.

79. Crispy Grilled Salmon Recipe

Serving: 6 | Prep: | Cook: 10mins | Ready in:

Ingredients

- 2 Pounds fresh salmon fillet, skin on
- 1 cup light cream
- 2 tbs. mayo
- salt and pepper
- 1 tsp. dried dill weed
- lemons
- Seasonings:
- 2 tbs peppercorn melody
- 1 tsp. coriander seed
- 1 tsp. dill seed
- 2 tsp. kosher salt

Direction

- Preheat grill
- Soak fish in cream for 30 minutes. Meanwhile place all the seasonings (only the seasonings under seasoning category) in a plastic bag and pound them with a mallet to crack them open. Remove fish from cream. Spread mayo on both sides of the fish. On the skin side season with salt and pepper. On the flesh side sprinkle with the dill weed and rub the crushed seasoning into the flesh. All the flesh should be covered with mayo and seasonings generously.
- Grill fish first seasoned side down 5-7 minutes, then 5-7 minutes on other side. Fish is done when it flakes with a fork. Remove and squeeze desired amount of lemon juice on it....and enjoy!

80. Crispy Tilapia With Avocado Pico De Gallo Recipe

Serving: 4 | Prep: | Cook: 12mins | Ready in:

Ingredients

- 1 firm avocado,chopped
- 1 cup purchased pico de gallo
- 1/4 cup chopped cilantro
- 1/2 cup yellow cornmeal
- 1/2 tsp ea. chili powder,ground cumin and salt
- 1/4 cup milk
- 11/2 lbs. tilapia fillets
- 3 Tbs oil
- corn on the cob

Direction

- Stir avocado into pico de gallo and cilantro; set aside. Mix cornmeal and chili powder, cumin and salt on sheet of waxed paper. Place milk in shallow bowl or pie plate. Dip tilapia fillets into milk, then cornmeal mixture to coat. Heat oil in large non-stick skillet over med. heat. Cook tilapia 2 to 3 mins a side. Top with avocado mixture; serve with corn on the cob.

81. Curried Cod In Coconut Broth Recipe

Serving: 4 | Prep: | Cook: 15mins | Ready in:

Ingredients

- 3 packs of ramen noodles, seasoning packet discarded
- 2 six ounce cod fillets (mine were frozen)
- 1 1/2 cups of chicken stock
- 8 ounces of coconut milk
- 1 tbsp. vegetable oil
- 1 red onion, cut in half moons
- 1 green pepper julienned
- 1 large garlic clove minced
- 3/4 cup of edamame, shelled
- 3/4 tsp. of curry powder
- 1/2 tsp. of cayenne pepper
- 1/2 tsp. turmeric
- 1/2 tsp. ginger
- 1/2 tsp. black pepper
- 1/2 tsp. salt
- generous red pepper flakes

Direction

- Break up the ramen noodles. Discard seasoning packets.
- Heat oil in deep sauté pan (I used my wok) and sauté onion, pepper strips and garlic until slightly softened.
- Add chicken broth and bring to a low boil.
- Add cod, seasonings/spices and ramen noodles.
- Simmer 5 minutes. Add coconut milk.
- Simmer another five minutes.
- Add edamame.
- Eat. Preferably with a cold beer to tame the heat.

82. Curried Cod With Tomato And Summer Squash Recipe

Serving: 2 | Prep: | Cook: 20mins | Ready in:

Ingredients

- 1 tb vegetable oil
- 1 1/2 tb curry paste
- 1 lb frozen cod; thawed
- 1/2 c chicken broth
- 2 ts fish sauce
- 1/2 onions; coarsely chopped
- 1 summer squash; seeded, chopped
- 1 tomatoes; seeded and chopped
- 1 tb fresh basil, chopped

Direction

- Heat oil in a wok or fry pan. Add curry paste and stir to soften.
- Add fresh fillets, cooking for about 1 minute on each side.
- Stir in chicken broth.
- Bring to a boil for 2 minutes

- Add summer squash and onions. Simmer on medium heat for 3 minutes.
- Add tomatoes and basil and steam until basil is just wilted, about 2-3 minutes.
- Serve immediately with Rice.

83. DEVILED SALMON CAKES Recipe

Serving: 4 | Prep: | Cook: 20mins | Ready in:

Ingredients

- 1 14 oz. can pink salmon, drained, skin and bones removed
- 2 Large eggs
- ½ cup diced sweet onion
- ½ cup diced yellow bell pepper (or any other color)
- 1 tsp minced garlic
- ½ tsp ground cumin
- ¼ to ½ tsp sea salt
- 1/8 to ¼ tsp ground cayenne pepper
- 2 cups cooked jasmine rice (or any sticky rice, leftover rice that will bind well)
- vegetable oil, or lard for frying - ¼ inch in frying pan or enough to cover half of your patty …I use lard…no apologies…

Direction

- Heat oil in skillet on Medium High heat.
- Mix salmon and rice together until thoroughly blended then add eggs.
- Add onion and pepper and mix well.
- Add spices.
- I use my hands and fingers to make sure everything is evenly distributed.
- When oil is hot form into patties in the palm of your hand.
- I made mine about 3 inches in diameter and not very thick (about the thickness of a hamburger patty)
- Place in hot oil and fry about 7 minutes on each side or until golden brown.
- When served fresh they are very crispy on the outside and moist on the inside.
- Awesome with Pinto Beans and Creamed Potatoes and skillet corn bread.
- Would also be great with a black bean and corn salsa.
- Serves 4 as main course or 12 as appetizers, depending on size of cake.

84. Dill Baked Salmon Recipe

Serving: 4 | Prep: | Cook: 20mins | Ready in:

Ingredients

- 1-1/2 pounds salmon steaks
- 1 teaspoon dill weed
- 1/2 teaspoon onion salt
- 1 lemon sliced

Direction

- Preheat oven to 425 then place salmon in baking dish sprayed with cooking spray.
- Sprinkle with dill and onion salt and top with lemon slices.
- Cover and bake 20 minutes.
- Serve with extra lemon.

85. Dill Haddock Recipe

Serving: 6 | Prep: | Cook: 12mins | Ready in:

Ingredients

- 6 fresh skinless haddock fillets
- 6 slices lemon
- 2 tablespoons snipped fresh dill
- 1 teaspoon freshly ground black pepper
- 1 teaspoon seasoned salt

Direction

- Rinse fish and pat dry then season with salt, pepper and dill.
- Place in a foil pouch then place slices of lemon on top of each fillet and seal bag.
- Place on grill for 6 minutes per side then remove to serving platter and serve immediately.

86. Earl Grey Salmon Recipe

Serving: 2 | Prep: | Cook: 10mins | Ready in:

Ingredients

- 2 6-ounce salmon steaks or fillets
- 3 ounces Earl Grey tea leaves
- 4 cups boiling water
- salt and pepper
- fresh lemon wedges (optional)

Direction

- Steep the tea in the boiling water for 10 minutes.
- Strain half of the tea leaves into a marinating container of some sort (with lid is great) and place the salmon pieces on top of the tea leaves.
- Strain the other half of the tea leaves on top of the salmon pieces.
- Spoon about 6 tbsps. of the steeped tea into the marinating container and cover.
- Marinate in the fridge for about 6 hours, turning the salmon pieces once or twice.
- The salmon can then be seasoned with salt and pepper and grilled, broiled or pan fried. A 6-ounce salmon fillet takes approximately 3 minutes per side to cook; a steak takes less than that, so watch carefully and don't overcook. It is cooked when it is no longer transparent in the middle.
- Serve with fresh lemon wedges. Anything else would mask the subtle flavour of the tea.

87. Easy Salmon Patties Recipe

Serving: 4 | Prep: | Cook: 10mins | Ready in:

Ingredients

- 1 15 oz. can red or pink salmon, bones removed
- 2 Tbs minced onion
- 1 Tbs. minced fresh parsley
- 1 large egg
- salt, pepper, dry dillweed to taste
- some fresh squeezed lemon juice
- Enough fresh bread crumbs to bind: try Japanese honey flavored panko breadcrumbs
- oil to sauté (peanut oil is nice)

Direction

- Combine everything and add enough breadcrumbs to bind mixture.
- Form into patties. These may be made ahead of time and chilled.
- Tip: chilling recommended so patties hold together better
- They fry in hot oil until golden on both sides. Turning carefully
- Serve with tartar sauce or mango mayo
- Note: by changing the herbs and spices (example add cilantro, ginger) one can easily change flavor

88. Easy Alaskan Salmon Teriyaki Bowl Recipe

Serving: 3 | Prep: | Cook: 15mins | Ready in:

Ingredients

- 1 (14.75-ounce) can Alaska salmon
- 1 cup instant or quick-cooking rice
- 1 tablespoon canola oil
- 1 (16-ounce) package frozen stir-fry vegetables

- 1/2 cup prepared thick teriyaki sauce
- 1/4 teaspoon red pepper flakes
- 1/4 teaspoon sesame oil
- 1/4 teaspoon ground ginger

Direction

- Prepare Rice according to package
- Drain salmon, dry and break into chunks, reserve 1 tablespoon of the liquid
- In a skillet or wok heat up the oil, and add veggies
- After about a minute add teriyaki sauce and salmon liquid and stir
- Add sesame oil, ginger, and red pepper flakes and salmon. Cook until vegetables are tender (about 3-5 minutes)
- Serve with rice

89. Easy Country Salmon Cakes Croquettes N Lemon Sauce Recipe

Serving: 4 | Prep: | Cook: 10mins | Ready in:

Ingredients

- Easy Country salmon cakes Croquettes n lemon Sauce
- 1 - 7 1/2 ounce can salmon, drained and flaked
- 1/3 cup of saltine cracker crumbs
- 1 egg, slightly beaten
- 2 tablespoons of chopped onion
- 2 tablespoons of milk
- 1 tablespoon of lemon juice
- 2 tablespoons butter or margarine
- In medium bowl, combine all ingredients except the butter, and blend well. Shape the mixture into 4 patties. Melt
- the butter in a skillet and fry the patties on both sides until golden brown and heated throughout
- lemon SAUCE:
- 1 c. lemon or orange juice
- 2 tbsp. cornstarch diluted in 1/4 c. cold water
- Bring all ingredients to a rolling boil in saucepan. Cook until sauce is clear. Serve hot over salmon croquettes.

Direction

- In medium bowl, combine all ingredients except the butter, and blend well.
- Shape the mixture into 4 patties.
- Melt the butter in a skillet and fry the patties on both sides until golden brown and heated throughout.
- LEMON SAUCE:
- 1 c. lemon or orange juice
- 2 tbsp. cornstarch diluted in 1/4 c. cold water
- Bring all ingredients to a rolling boil in saucepan. Cook until sauce is clear. Serve hot over or with salmon croquettes.

90. Easy Delicious Poached Salmon In Crock Pot Recipe

Serving: 4 | Prep: | Cook: 180mins | Ready in:

Ingredients

- 4 salmon fillets (could be salmon steaks)
- 1/2 pint water
- 1/4 pint white wine
- 1 tsp salt
- 2 bay leaves
- 2 peppercorns
- 1 sprig fresh rosemary
- Few springs of fresh oregano or thyme
- 1 small onion sliced into thin circles
- 1 Fresh lemon sliced (garnish)
- fresh parsley (garnish)

Direction

- Lightly oil the bottom of the slow cooker and place the salmon evenly on the bottom. Heat remaining ingredients to a near boil.
- Pour over the salmon in crock pot.

- Cover and cook low for approximately 3 hours or until salmon is cooked and done.
- Carefully remove salmon.
- Garnish with fresh chopped parsley and lemon slices.
- Yield: 2 to 4 servings.

91. Easy Grilled TROUT Recipe

Serving: 1 | Prep: | Cook: 15mins | Ready in:

Ingredients

- 1 fresh trout (entrails removed)
- butter (your preference of amount)
- ==================================
- Seasoning:
- lemon slices
- lime slices
- 1/2 tsp oregano
- 1 sprig rosemary
- Minced garlic (optional)
- salt and pepper to preference

Direction

- Preparation:
- Place one headless trout on a sheet of aluminum foil.
- Insert several slices of butter, lemon and lime, and herbs inside the trout.
- Add minced garlic if desired.
- Wrap trout in foil so it's sealed, like a neat package.
- Cook trout over hot coals or an open flame for approximately 5-7 minutes on each side, cooking time will vary depending on temperature of the grill.
- Remove from heat.
- Open foil and allow several minutes to cool.
- Hold trout and flake off one side fillet from bone.
- Turn trout over and repeat.
- All bones should be removed by using this method.

92. Easy Roast Salmon With Veggies Recipe

Serving: 3 | Prep: | Cook: 35mins | Ready in:

Ingredients

- 3 salmon steaks
- 9 onions
- 3 carrots
- 1 c. marinated mushrooms
- 1/2 c. olive oil
- glass of water
- juice of 1 lemon
- salt
- pepper
- 2 tblsp Trinidad hot sauce
- oregano

Direction

- Place the 3 salmon steaks on the tray
- Cut the 9 onions in halves place face down around the steaks, together with three carrots sliced in half across the center, and a cup of marinated mushrooms.
- pour half a cup of Olive Oil, a glass of water, the juice of one lemon, salt and pepper, 2 tablespoons of Trinidad Hot Sauce and a pinch of oregano over the salmon
- Cover the tray with foil and bake for 30 minutes at 375 degrees. When just about ready turn the salmon upside down
- Separate the layers of the onions and bake a little bit more until the water evaporates and the steaks are a golden colour

93. Easy, Perfect Baked Haddock Recipe

Serving: 4 | Prep: | Cook: 25mins | Ready in:

Ingredients

- 4 haddock fillets,cleaned,rinsed and pat dry
- 1/2 stick butter ,melted
- 3/4 roll Ritz crackers,crushed
- dash of black pepper or lemon pepper
- 1 TB(1/3 squeezed)lemon juice to taste
- 1/2 tsp dried or fresh parsley

Direction

- Preheat oven to 350.
- Melt butter in small glass bowl, add Ritz cracker crumbs and combine gently. Spray shallow baking pan with spray, put few cracker crumbs in bottom of pan. Lay haddock in pan, cover with remaining cracker crumbs, squeeze lemon and sprinkle parsley over fish.
- Bake 350° for 10-20 mins, watching closely, as fillets vary in size, don't overcook! Mine took 12 mins, I put under broiler for a min or two to crisp up a little more. Remove when fish is white and flakes easily.

94. Elaines HEALTHY Salmon Tortilla Wraps Recipe

Serving: 2 | Prep: | Cook: | Ready in:

Ingredients

- 1 can red salmon
- butter for spreading
- 1 whole lemon, peeled and cut thinly into slices
- 2 green onions, finely chopped
- 1 baby red onion, finely chopped
- 1 tbsp Zesty Italian salad dressing
- 2 large leaves romaine lettuce, trimmed of center leaf vein
- 2 10 inch tortillas, whole wheat

Direction

- Butter the tortillas
- Add to the salmon:
- The onions
- The salad dressing
- Combine well.
- Spread the salmon over the tortilla, leaving about 1 inch free space around the edges. This makes it easier to roll, and eliminates spill over.
- Now, add three thin slices of fresh lemon
- Add the trimmed Romaine lettuce
- Roll the tortilla into a neat, tight bundle.
- Refrigerate until ready to use, or serve immediately.
- Delicious

95. Elaines Steelhead Salmon HEART HEALTHY Bake With French Brandy Sauce Recipe

Serving: 2 | Prep: | Cook: 25mins | Ready in:

Ingredients

- 1 lb full side Steelhead salmon fillet
- 2 lemons, sliced - peel on
- 1 tbsp olive oil
- ¼ tsp salt
- 1.4 tsp pepper
- 1 tbsp balsamic vinegar
- ==================================
- For the Sauce:
- 2 oz French brandy
- 2 oz lemon juice
- 3 tsp raw sugar
- 1 tsp pure vanilla extract

Direction

- Cover a baking sheet with tinfoil
- Place on the foil slices of lemon, enough to lay out the salmon on
- Salt & pepper as desired (keeping in mind the heart-healthy aims...!)
- Drizzle with olive oil & Balsamic vinegar

- Place more lemon slices on top
- Bake, covered with foil, until fish is tender, and flakes easily.
- The Sauce:
- Combine the Brandy, lemon juice, sugar, and vanilla
- Reduce at medium-high heat until ½ original quantity.
- Drizzle over or around fish
- Serve with VEG MEDLEY, separately posted.
- (I served the fish on top of the vegetable medley, the two dishes marry so well!)

96. FIRECRACKER SALMON STEAKS Recipe

Serving: 4 | Prep: | Cook: 20mins | Ready in:

Ingredients

- Ingredients:
- ¼ cup balsamic vinegar
- ¼ cup chili sauce
- ¼ cup packed brown sugar
- 3 garlic cloves, minced
- 2 tsp. Minced fresh parsley
- ¼ tsp. ground ginger or 1tsp. Minced fresh gingerroot
- ¼ to ½ tsp. cayenne pepper
- ¼ to ½ tsp. crushed red pepper flakes, optional
- 4 salmon steaks (6-oz each)

Direction

- In a small bowl, combine the first 8 ingredients. If grilling the salmon, coat grilling rack with non-stick cooking spray before starting the grill. Grill salmon, un-covered, over medium heat or broil 4 - 6-inches from the heat for 4 - 5 minutes on each side or until fish flakes easily with a fork, brushing occasionally with sauce.
- Serving size: 1 steak
- Nutrition Values: Calories per serving: 373, Fat: 17g, Cholesterol: 106mg, Sodium: 565mg, Carbohydrate: 22g, Protein: 32g
- Diabetic Exchanges: 5 lean meat, 1 ½ starch
- NOTE: This recipe is Diabetic Friendly, Gastric Bypass friendly, and for anyone.

97. Fabulous Salmon Provencal Recipe

Serving: 4 | Prep: | Cook: 12mins | Ready in:

Ingredients

- Here's a salmon dish made for summer.
- salmon Provencal Recipe
- 3 large plum tomatoes
- 3 shallots, coarsely chopped
- 1 Tbsp coarsely chopped fresh tarragon
- 1 Tbsp coarsely chopped fresh basil
- 1 Tbsp coarsely chopped fresh chives
- 1 Tbsp fresh lemon juice
- 1 Tbsp balsamic vinegar
- salt
- 2 Tbsp olive oil
- 4 salmon fillets, about 5-6 ounces each

Direction

- Preheat oven to 400°F.
- Blanch the tomatoes by plunging them into a pot of simmering salted water for 15-30 seconds, then plunging them into ice water for 1 minute. Drain the tomatoes and peel off and discard the skin. Cut the tomatoes into quarters, remove the core, seeds, and dice the flesh.
- In a large bowl combine the tomatoes, shallots, tarragon, basil, and chives. In another bowl, whisk together the lemon juice, vinegar, olive oil and salt to taste. Add to the tomato mixture, toss to coat.
- Arrange salmon fillets on an oiled baking sheet without crowding. Drizzle with olive oil and season lightly with salt. Bake until salmon

is barely cooked through and lightly browned on the edges, 10-12 minutes.

- To serve, spoon a couple tablespoons of the tomato mixture over each fillet. Serve immediately.

98. Fast And Easy Haddock Au Gratin Recipe

Serving: 6 | Prep: | Cook: 15mins | Ready in:

Ingredients

- 1 1/2 to 2 pound haddock fillets or other firm white fish
- 1 can cream of cream of celery soup (I used reduced sodium)
- 1/2 cup milk
- 2 Tbsp. sherry
- 1/2 cup shredded mild cheddar cheese
- 1 1/2 cups bread crumbs tossed with 3 tablespoons melted butter
- 1 Tbsp. fresh parsley

Direction

- Arrange haddock in a shallow buttered baking dish. Combine soup with milk in a saucepan over medium low heat and heat through. Add sherry and stir to combine. Pour soup mixture over the fish. Sprinkle with shredded cheese. Combine parsley and buttered bread crumbs. Bake for 10 to 15 minutes, or until golden on top and fish is flaky and cooked through.

99. Fennel And Peppercorn Crusted Tuna Steaks Recipe

Serving: 2 | Prep: | Cook: 20mins | Ready in:

Ingredients

- 1 tbsp fennel seeds
- 1 tbsp peppercorns
- 1 tsp dried rosemary
- 1/4 tsp crushed red pepper flakes
- 2 cloves garlic
- 1/2 tsp kosher salt
- 2 tuna steaks
- 2 tbsp. olive oil

Direction

- Crush fennel seeds, peppercorns, pepper flakes and dried rosemary in a mortar and pestle (or pulse once or twice in a spice grinder - you want them slightly ground, but not pulverized).
- Add garlic and salt, if using mortar and pestle, and smash until garlic is evenly distributed (will look like consistency of wet sand, not paste-like). If you used the spice grinder, coarsely chop garlic and leave on cutting board. Sprinkle with spice mixture and salt and press into with the side of a knife or bottom of pan until blended.
- Rinse tuna steaks and pat dry; press garlic-spice mixture into both sides of steaks.
- Place dry skillet over medium-high heat - let pan get hot. Gently place tuna steaks in pan.
- Cook about 2-3 minutes on each side for rare, 3-4 for medium (my preference!), carefully flipping with spatula. Just like with steak, it will "tell" you when it's ready to flip - when it's seared properly, the tuna will no longer stick to the pan.
- Remove from heat and cover for about 5 minutes.
- You can serve as is or slice into 1/2" slices.

100. Fish Filets With Bacon And Horseradish Recipe

Serving: 6 | Prep: | Cook: 30mins | Ready in:

Ingredients

- 8 firm flesh white fish filets (cod, haddock, pollock, catfish)
- 2 tablespoons butter
- 1/4 cup sweet onion, chopped
- 1 (8 ounce) package cream cheese, softened
- 1/4 cup dry white wine
- 2 tablespoons prepared horseradish
- 1 tablespoon Dijon mustard
- 1/2 teaspoon salt, or to taste
- 1/8 teaspoon ground black pepper
- 4 strips bacon, cooked and crumbled
- 2 tablespoons fresh parsley, minced

Direction

- Rinse fish filets and pat dry. Arrange in large baking dish in a single layer.
- In small skillet, melt butter over medium-high heat. Add onion and sauté until softened.
- Combine cream cheese, wine, horseradish, mustard, salt and pepper. Stir into onion in skillet.
- Pour mixture over fish. Top with crumbled bacon.
- Bake at 350 degrees for 30 minutes or until fish flakes easily.
- Garnish with parsley.
- I like to serve the filets on a bed of sautéed fresh spinach.

101. Fish Filets With Lemon Caper Sauce Recipe

Serving: 4 | Prep: | Cook: | Ready in:

Ingredients

- For fish preparation:
- 8 large mushrooms, sautéed in a little butter
- 4 mild white fish fillets, such as tilapia
- 1 tablespoon (or less) butter, for skillet
- 1 cup white wine
- ¼ teaspoon salt
- dash of pepper
- 1 tablespoon capers
- Sauce:
- 3 tablespoons butter
- 1 tablespoon flour
- 2 egg yolks
- ½ cup half-and-half
- ¼ cup reserved liquid from fish prep skillet
- salt and pepper, to taste
- 1 tablespoon fresh lemon juice, or to your taste
- lemon wedges for garnish

Direction

- In a large skillet, sauté mushrooms in some butter; remove them from the pan and place fish fillets in the pan with a bit more butter.
- Add wine, salt, pepper and capers.
- Bring to boil, reduce heat, cover and simmer gently for 10 minutes (while fish is simmering, begin sauce preparation).
- Remove fish to serving platter, top with sautéed mushrooms.
- Keep fish warm (I put mine on a cookie sheet, cover it with foil, and keep warm in a 250 degree oven).
- Cook remaining liquid in pan until it is reduced to ½ cup; strain and reserve ¼ cup for sauce (I like capers, so I do not strain my liquid - I just use it all and increase the flour in the sauce by about a 1/2 tablespoon).
- For sauce, melt butter in a saucepan and stir in flour.
- Simmer very gently for 3 minutes.
- Stir together yolks and cream; add reserved liquid from skillet and stir into flour mixture.
- Season to taste.
- Add lemon juice.
- Pour sauce over warm fish and mushrooms.
- Garnish with lemon wedges

102. Fish In Tomato Rhubarb N Blood Orange Sauce Recipe

Serving: 8 | Prep: | Cook: 65mins | Ready in:

Ingredients

- For the sauce
- 3 medium blood oranges (or 2 large, juicy navel oranges)
- 2 tablespoons olive oil
- 2 cups finely chopped onion
- 1 1/2 teaspoons fresh ginger, peeled and finely minced
- 1 tablespoon honey, orange blossom or other light floral flavor
- salt and freshly ground black pepper
- 1 pound rhubarb, ends trimmed (discard leaves, which can be toxic), tough strings removed with a vegetable peeler, and stalks cut into 1-inch pieces (4 cups)
- 1 cup fresh orange juice
- Generous pinch of ground cinnamon
- 2 cups canned, peeled plum tomatoes (about a pound), coarsely chopped, and 1/2 cup of their liquid.
- juice of 1/2 lemon
- -----------------
- For the fish
- ----------------
- 3 pounds fish fillets or steaks (salmon, red snapper, grouper, sea bass, halibut, cod or sole)
- 1/3 to 1/2 cup mint leaves, finely minced for garnish

Direction

- Make the sauce

103. Fish N Chips Recipe

Serving: 0 | Prep: | Cook: 35mins | Ready in:

Ingredients

- frying oil (I use peanut) about 8 cups
- 4-8 pieces cod or similar type fish
- 1 cup flour
- 1/4 tsp salt
- 1 egg
- 1 Tbsp melted butter
- 2/3 cup milk
- 6-8 large regular potatoes cut up
- malt vinegar

Direction

- I use an electric deep fryer with a thermometer attached. Heat oil to about 350 deg. Mix together flour, salt, egg, butter and milk (can use buttermilk) well. Dip fish pieces and coat well with thick batter, then put into the hot oil. I do not use the basket for these as they stick. Cook about 5 minutes for small pieces, 8 for larger. Drizzle in the left over batter for cracking. Use tongs to transfer cooked fish to a paper towel to drain. You can keep fish warm in a warm oven while you do the chips.
- I use the basket for the chips. Put potato pieces into the basket and into the hot oil and cook 10-15 minutes or until done. Drain and transfer to paper towel to drain. Serve with Malt Vinegar.

104. Fish Veracruzana Recipe

Serving: 4 | Prep: | Cook: 25mins | Ready in:

Ingredients

- 1 lb fish - scrod, catfish, flounder - cut in chunks
- 3 large new potatoes, scrubbed (not peeled) and cut in half
- 3 T oil
- 2 medium onions, sliced thin
- 2 bell peppers (any color), seeded and sliced
- 2 anaheim or 1 poblano chili, seeded and sliced (I use a dash of hot sauce instead)
- 1/2 cup white wine
- 4 T lime juice
- 2 tsp minced garlic
- 1 1/2 cup tomato puree or diced tomatoes
- 1 bunch cilantro (optional)

Direction

- Put potatoes through the thick blade of a food processor.
- Heat oil in an extra large skillet.
- Sauté onions until translucent, then move them to the side and add potatoes
- Cook, stirring often, until the potatoes take on color
- Add peppers, chilies, and lime juice.
- Cook until the potatoes soften, about 15 minutes.
- Add half of cilantro leaves (if using), tomatoes, and fish.
- Cover fish with vegetables.
- Cook 8 minutes, until fish is done.
- Serve with remaining cilantro and lime wedges for garnish.

105. Fish With Leeks And Fermented Soy Beans Recipe

Serving: 2 | Prep: | Cook: 15mins | Ready in:

Ingredients

- 1 tilapia fish
- 1 stalk green onions (cut into 2" lengths)
- 4-5 slices ginger
- 1 stalk leeks (use 2 stalks if you love leeks) (cut the white part into slices on the bias)
- 1/4 lb minced pork (the non-lean type)
- 1 tbsp fermented soy beans
- 1/2 bowl warm water
- 1 tsp sugar
- 2 red chillies (remove seeds and cut into slices)
- corn starch water

Direction

- Season minced pork with a sprinkle of salt, a couple dashes of white pepper and a sprinkle of corn starch. Mix well.
- Do the same for the tilapia. Sprinkle salt, white pepper and corn starch on the inside (stomach) and outside (skin) and gently rub the seasoning onto the tilapia. Insert 2-3 slices of ginger and a few pieces of spring onions into the stomach of the tilapia.
- Heat up 3-4 tbsp oil in a wok. Pan-fry fish until both sides become golden brown or cooked. Dish out and set aside.
- In the same wok, add the remaining green onions and ginger. Add the minced pork and stir fry until fragrant before adding the leeks. Fry over high heat until fragrant, then add the fermented soy beans and mix well.
- Add in the tilapia and half a bowl of water and cook over low heat for about 10 mins. (Cover wok so that the gravy won't evaporate.)
- Add sugar and chili slices and mix well. Slowly add corn starch solution and stir well until desired gravy thickness.
- Serve the Fish with leeks and fermented soy beans with plain white rice and remember to drizzle the flavorful gravy over the rice. Enjoy!

106. Flounder Jardiniere Recipe

Serving: 6 | Prep: | Cook: 25mins | Ready in:

Ingredients

- 1/3 cup all-purpose flour
- 3 eggs, lightly beaten
- 2 tablespoons butter
- 2 tablespoons oil
- 6 fillet (about 1-3/4 pounds)
- 1 leek, cut in 2-inch pieces, thinly sliced lengthwise
- 3 carrots, cut in 2-inch pieces, thinly sliced lengthwise
- 1/4 teaspoon salt
- 1/8 teaspoon pepper
- 3/4 cup chicken broth
- 1/4 cup dry white wine
- 1 tablespoon fresh lemon juice
- 3 tablespoons capers, drained

Direction

- Place flour in small pan; place eggs in small bowl.
- Heat half the butter and oil in large nonstick skillet.
- Coat 3 fillets with flour; dip in eggs. Cook in skillet 2-1/2 minutes per side, until lightly golden.
- Remove to platter; keep warm. Add remaining butter and oil to skillet. Cook remaining fillets.
- To skillet, add leek, carrots, salt and pepper; sauté 4 minutes; if dry, add more butter.
- Add broth, wine, lemon and capers.
- Cover; cook 6 minutes, until carrots are tender. Spoon over fish.
- Makes 6 servings.

107. Flounder With Tomato Onion Ragout Recipe

Serving: 1 | Prep: | Cook: 25mins | Ready in:

Ingredients

- 1-½ teaspoons olive oil
- ¼ medium red onion, thinly sliced
- ½ cup grape or cherry tomatoes, halved
- 1 to 2 teaspoons white-wine vinegar
- coarse salt and ground pepper
- 1 flounder fillet (5 to 6 ounces)
- 2 tablespoons chopped fresh parsley

Direction

- Tomato-onion ragout:
- In a 10-inch skillet, heat ½ teaspoon oil over medium. Add onion and cook, stirring occasionally, until light browned, 1 to 2 minutes. Add tomatoes and cook, stirring occasionally, until slightly collapsed, 30 to 60 seconds.
- Remove skillet from heat. Add vinegar; stir to combine. Season with salt and pepper. Remove to a bowl; cover and keep warm.
- Flounder:
- Wipe skillet clean with paper towels. Place 1 teaspoon oil in pan, and heat over medium-high. Season fish with salt and pepper; place in skillet. Cook, until lightly browned, about 2 minutes.
- With a wide metal spatula, carefully turn fish over; cook until opaque throughout, about 1 minute. Transfer fish to a dinner plate. Spoon tomato-onion ragout over fish; serve with couscous or rice, if desired. Sprinkle parsley over top.

108. Fresh Fillet Of Sole With Lemon Cream Recipe

Serving: 4 | Prep: | Cook: 6mins | Ready in:

Ingredients

- 2 tablespoons butter
- 2 pounds sole fillets, cut to make 4 pieces
- 3/4 teaspoon salt
- 1/4 teaspoon fresh-ground black pepper
- 1/4 cup flour
- 3/4 cup heavy cream
- Grated zest of 1/2 lemon
- 1 tablespoon lemon juice
- 2 tablespoons chopped fresh parsley

Direction

- In a large nonstick frying pan, melt the butter over moderate heat. Sprinkle the sole with 1/2 teaspoon of the salt and the pepper. Dust the sole with the flour and shake off any excess. Put the sole in the pan and cook for 2 minutes. Turn and cook until just done, about 2 minutes longer. Remove the sole from the pan.
- Add the cream and lemon zest to the pan. Bring to a simmer and cook until starting to thicken, about 2 minutes. Stir in the remaining 1/4 teaspoon salt, the lemon juice, and parsley. Serve the sauce over the fish.

- Fish Alternatives: Other members of the flounder family, such as sand dab or fluke, will go well with the sauce, as will such mild fish fillets as trout, hake, or whiting.
- Wine Recommendation: A ripe, full-flavored chardonnay with oak overtones will be well suited to the richness of this creamy dish. Try a bottle from California or Australia.

109. Garam Masala Seared Salmon With A Coconut Curry Butter Recipe

Serving: 8 | Prep: | Cook: 25mins | Ready in:

Ingredients

- 8 ea., 7 oz. salmon fillets
- 2 Tbsp. prepared garam masala spice mixture
- kosher salt to taste
- 3-4 Tbsp. oil for frying
- For the sauce:
- 3/4 c. dry white wine
- 1/3 c. heavy cream
- 2/3 c. Premium unsweetened coconut milk
- 2 Tbsp. Indian curry powder
- 2 bay leaves
- 3-4 cloves
- 1 c. cold unsalted butter, cut into small cubes
- kosher salt to taste

Direction

- In a saucepan, combine all of the ingredients for the sauce except for the butter and salt. Bring to light boil, then reduce to a simmer and cook until the sauce reduces to 1/2 cup. Turn the heat down to low, then whisk in the butter until it is incorporated into the sauce. Do NOT let the sauce boil at this point. Season to taste and reserve.
- Keep the sauce warm.
- Pre-heat oven to 400 F. In an oven proof sauté pan or heavy skillet, heat the oil until lightly smoking. Season both sides of the fish with salt and sprinkle with the garam-masala. Pan sear for approximately 1 minute per side, then finish cooking in the oven for about 6-7 minutes, or until desired doneness is achieved. Serve immediately with the coconut-curry butter.

110. Garlic And Herb Crusted Mahi Mahi With Salsa Recipe

Serving: 4 | Prep: | Cook: 20mins | Ready in:

Ingredients

- 1 cup seeded and diced Japanese cucumber
- 1/2 cup seeded and diced red tomato
- 3 yellow pear tomatoes cut in half
- 2 tablespoons finely minced ginger
- 1/4 cup finely minced onion
- 2 tablespoons soy sauce
- 2 tablespoons spicy sesame oil
- 1/2 teaspoon salt
- 1 teaspoon freshly ground black pepper
- garlic herb Crust:
- 1/4 cup coarsely chopped garlic
- 1 teaspoon chopped fresh parsley
- 1 tablespoon chopped fresh basil
- 1 teaspoon chopped fresh tarragon
- 4 anchovy fillets
- 4 shallots roughly chopped
- 1 teaspoon virgin olive oil
- 4 mahi mahi fillets
- 1 teaspoon canola oil

Direction

- Combine all salsa ingredients in mixing bowl and stir until well combined then chill.
- Place all crust ingredients in a food processor or blender and puree.
- Coat one side of each fillet with crust and allow to sit 15 minutes.

- Heat canola in non-stick sauté pan and sear crusted fillets over high heat for 1 minute per side.
- Place fish crust side up on 4 serving plates and spoon salsa over and around each serving.

111. Gas Grill Red Snapper Recipe

Serving: 4 | Prep: | Cook: 8mins | Ready in:

Ingredients

- 2Tbs. sweet paprika
- 2tsp onion powder
- 2tsp garlic powder
- 3/4tsp ground coriander
- 3/4tsp table salt
- 1/4tsp cayenne pepper
- 1/4tsp black pepper
- 1/4tsp white pepper
- 2Tbs unsalted butter
- Large aluminum disposable baking pan
- 4 red snapper fillets,6-8oz. each,3/4" thick
- veg. oil for grill rack

Direction

- Combine paprika, onion powder, garlic powder, ground coriander, salt and peppers in small bowl. Melt butter in 10" skillet over med. heat. When foaming subsides, stir in spice mixture. Cook, stirring frequently, till fragrant and spices turn a dark rust color, 2-3 mins. Transfer mixture to pie plate and cool, stirring occasionally, to room temp., about 10 mins. Once cooled, use fork to break any clumps.
- Turn all burners to high, cover, and heat grill till very hot, about 15 mins. Use grill brush to scrape clean.
- Meanwhile, pat fillets dry on both sides with paper towels. Using sharp knife, make shallow diagonal slashes every inch along skin side of fish, being careful not to cut flesh. Place fillets skin side up on rimmed baking sheet. Using fingers, rub spice mixture in thin even layers on top and side of fish. Flip fillets over and repeat on other side (use all spice mixture). Refrigerate till needed.
- Lightly dip wad of paper towel in oil; holding with tongs, wipe cooking grate. Place fish perpendicular to grill grates, skin side down on grill. Leaving burners on high, grill uncovered until very dark brown and skin crisp, 3-4 mins. Using thin metal spatula, flip fish and continue to grill till dark brown, beginning to flake, and center is opaque but still moist, about 5 mins longer.
- This is great with remoulade sauce or pineapple or mango salsa.

112. Gingered Salmon In Carrot And Orange Sauce Recipe

Serving: 4 | Prep: | Cook: 15mins | Ready in:

Ingredients

- 1.5 lb salmon fillet skinned and without bones
- 1 + 1/4 cups fresh carrot juice*
- 1/2 cup (minus 1 Tbsp) freshly squeezed orange juice
- Juice of 1/2 lemon
- 1/2 cup butter, cold
- 3 inch fresh ginger root
- 3 scallions
- 1/4 cup unsalted peanuts, coarsely chopped
- 1 Tbsp canola oil
- 1 Tbsp olive oil
- A dash of cayenne pepper
- Fleur de sel (or seasalt)
- 2 cups cleaned snow peas, or sugar snap peas and rice to accompany
- 1 cup bean sprouts to garnish
- Note
- ——
- It's advised that you make your own fresh carrot juice if you have a juicer (mine is the

Juiceman Juicer), it is so much better. You will never go back to store-bought carrot juice!

Direction

- To prepare the sauce, start by slicing half of the ginger in small pieces.
- Pour the carrot juice in a small pot with the slices of ginger.
- Bring to a light boil, then simmer and cook until the juice is reduced by half.
- Add the orange juice and repeat the process.
- Remove from the heat and take out the ginger slices.
- Add the cold butter in small pieces mixing with a whip and add the lemon juice. Keep warm on the side.
- To prepare the garnish, start by cleaning the scallions. Cut them in diagonal. Blanch them in salted boiling water for 2 min. Remove and strain on paper towels.
- Chop the nuts coarsely and chop the ginger thinly.
- Mix all ingredients with 1 Tbsp. canola oil and keep on the side.
- To prepare the fish, dice the salmon in one inch squares.
- Heat 1 to 2 Tbsp. of olive oil in a non-stick frying pan. When the oil is hot, add the pieces of fish and cook lightly for 1 min on one side, then on the other. Do not overcook the fish as it should actually stay rosé, that is a little undercooked.
- Add a pinch of cayenne pepper.
- To assemble your dish, take warm plates and place some fish pieces in the middle. Pour some orange sauce around.
- Sprinkle with fleur de sel (sea salt) and add the peanut/scallions mixture on top.
- Serve with jasmine rice and steamed snow (or sugar snap) peas.

113. Gnocchi With A Gorgonzola And Smoked Salmon Sauce Recipe

Serving: 4 | Prep: | Cook: 25mins | Ready in:

Ingredients

- 30ML butter
- 180G gorgonzola, CRUMBLED
- PINCH ground nutmeg
- 45ML brandy (OPTIONAL)
- 190ML chicken stock
- 250 CREAM
- 500G READY-MADE gnocchi
- olive oil, FOR DRIZZLING
- 100G smoked salmon, SLICED
- PARMESON cheese AND fresh herbs, TO SERVE

Direction

- MELT THE BUTTER IN A LARGE POT
- ADD THE GORGONZOLA CHEESE AND STIR UNTIL IT HAS MELTED
- ADD THE NUTMEG, BRANDY AND THE CHICKEN STOCK, THEN WHISK IN THE CREAM
- BRING TO THE BOIL
- PLACE THE GNOCCHI IN A LARGE PAN AND DREIZZLE WITH OLIVE OIL
- COVER WITH A LID AND COOK UNTIL SOFT IN THE CENTRE
- REMOVE THE LID AND FRYN UNTIL CRISP AND GOLDEN
- ADD THE SALMON TO THE SAUCE AND LEAVE IT TO SIMMER FOR TWO MINUTES
- POUR A LITTLE SAUCE INTO EACH DISH AND TOP WITH GNOCCHI
- SEASON TO TASTE WITH SALT (BE CAREFUL WITH THE SALT) AND FRESHLY GROUND BLACK PEPPER AND GARNISH WITH PARMESAN SHAVINGS AND HERS.
- ENJOY!

114. Godeungeo Jorim (braised Mackerel) Recipe

Serving: 4 | Prep: | Cook: 50mins | Ready in:

Ingredients

- •2 mackerel, de-gutted & cleaned
- •2 tbsp gochugaru (Korean red pepper flakes)
- •1 tbsp gochujang (Korean red pepper paste)
- •2 tbsp cooking wine (or mirin)
- •2 tbsp soy sauce
- •1 tbsp brown sugar
- •5 garlic cloves, minced
- •1/2 tsp ginger, minced
- •2 green onions
- •2 hot pepper (red and green each; optional)
- •2 cups water
- •4 anchovies (optional; broth)

Direction

- 1. Cut the radish into semi-circular pieces about a half-inch thick. Prepare other sauce ingredients and combine in a mixing bowl.
- 2. In a pot, add 2 cups of water and sliced radish. Bring water to a boil for about 10 minutes.
- 3. After degutting and cleaning the mackerel well under cold water, cut mackerel into 3-inch pieces. Add to the pot of boiling water.
- 4. Pour the sauce on top of the mackerel. Boil until the soup has reduced to half. Do not stir the mixture, but coat the sauce over the top of the mackerel carefully. Cook on high for 10 minutes and then let simmer. Keep lid semi-closed allowing the sauce to thicken over time.
- 5. After simmering about 15 minutes, add the scallions.
- 6. Serve with rice and other side dishes.

115. Golden Halibut Puffs Recipe

Serving: 4 | Prep: | Cook: 15mins | Ready in:

Ingredients

- 16 ounces frozen halibut fillets thawed
- 1 teaspoon salt
- 1 teaspoon freshly ground black pepper
- 1 egg white
- 1/8 teaspoon salt
- 1/4 cup mayonnaise
- 1/4 teaspoon dill seed
- 1/4 teaspoon onion juice

Direction

- Preheat oven to 425.
- Place fillets in greased baking dish and season with salt and pepper.
- Beat egg white and salt until stiff but not dry.
- Fold in remaining ingredients and spoon onto fish.
- Bake uncovered 15 minutes or until fish flakes easily with fork and topping puffed and brown.

116. Grilled Catfish Tacos With Citrus Slaw Recipe

Serving: 4 | Prep: | Cook: 15mins | Ready in:

Ingredients

- 4 catfish fillets
- 1 tablespoon mild or hot chili powder
- 1 tablespoon canola oil
- 1 tablespoon fresh lemon or lime juice
- 4 flour tortillas, "soft taco" (10-inch) size
- Lemon and/or lime wedges
- Citrus Slaw
- 2 cups finely shredded cabbage
- 2 TBS orange juice concentrate (do not dilute)
- 1/2 cup thinly sliced green bell pepper

- 1/2 cup thinly sliced onion
- 2 tablespoons canola oil
- 2 tablespoons apple cider vinegar

Direction

- 1. Prepare grill. Combine chili powder, oil and lemon juice in a small bowl; brush over both sides of fillets. Arrange in a wire-grilling basket coated with cooking spray.
- 2. Place grilling basket on a grill rack; grill 6-8 minutes on each side until catfish flakes easily when tested with a fork. Place 1 fillet on a tortilla, and top with ¾ cup Citrus Slaw. 3. For Citrus Slaw: Combine all ingredients in a bowl; tossing gently. Cover and chill.

117. Grilled Cilantro Salmon Recipe

Serving: 4 | Prep: | Cook: 20mins | Ready in:

Ingredients

- 1 bunch cilantro leaves, chopped
- 2 cloves garlic, chopped
- 2 cups honey
- juice from one lime
- 4 salmon steaks
- salt and pepper to taste

Direction

- 1. In a saucepan over medium-low heat, stir together cilantro, garlic, honey, and lime juice. Heat until the honey is easily stirred, about 5 minutes. Remove from heat, and let cool slightly.
- 2. Place salmon steaks in a baking dish, and season with salt and pepper. Pour marinade over salmon, cover, and refrigerate 10 minutes.
- 3. Preheat grill for high heat. Lightly oil grill grate. Place salmon steaks on grill, cook 5-to 6 minutes on each side, or until fish is easily flaked with a fork.

118. Grilled Fish Taco With Chipotle Lime Dressing Recipe

Serving: 6 | Prep: | Cook: 9mins | Ready in:

Ingredients

- marinade
- 1/4 cup extra virgin olive oil
- 2 tablespoons distilled white vinegar
- 2 tablespoons fresh lime juice
- 2 teaspoons lime zest
- 1 1/2 teaspoons honey
- 2 cloves garlic, minced
- 1/2 teaspoon cumin
- 1/2 teaspoon chili powder
- 1 teaspoon seafood seasoning, such as Old Bay™
- 1/2 teaspoon ground black pepper
- 1 teaspoon hot pepper sauce, or to taste
- 1 pound tilapia fillets, cut into chunks
- Dressing
- 1 (8 ounce) container light sour cream
- 1/2 cup adobo sauce from chipotle peppers
- 2 tablespoons fresh lime juice
- 2 teaspoons lime zest
- 1/4 teaspoon cumin
- 1/4 teaspoon chili powder
- 1/2 teaspoon seafood seasoning, such as Old Bay™
- salt and pepper to taste
- Toppings
- 1 (10 ounce) package tortillas
- 3 ripe tomatoes, seeded and diced
- 1 bunch cilantro, chopped
- 1 small head cabbage, cored and shredded
- 2 limes, cut in wedges

Direction

- To make the marinade, whisk together the olive oil, vinegar, lime juice, lime zest, honey, garlic, cumin, chili powder, seafood seasoning, black pepper, and hot sauce in a bowl until blended. Place the tilapia in a shallow dish, and pour the marinade over the fish.

- Cover, and refrigerate 6 to 8 hours.
- To make the dressing, combine the sour cream and adobo sauce in a bowl.
- Stir in the lime juice, lime zest, cumin, chili powder, seafood seasoning.
- Add salt, and pepper in desired amounts.
- Cover, and refrigerate until needed.
- Preheat an outdoor grill for high heat and lightly oil grate. Set grate 4 inches from the heat.
- Remove fish from marinade, drain off any excess and discard marinade.
- Grill fish pieces until easily flaked with a fork, turning once, about 9 minutes.
- Assemble tacos by placing fish pieces in the center of tortillas with desired amounts of tomatoes, cilantro, and cabbage; drizzle with dressing.
- To serve, roll up tortillas around fillings, and garnish with lime wedges.

119. Grilled Fish Tacos Recipe

Serving: 6 | Prep: | Cook: 8mins | Ready in:

Ingredients

- 2 pounds fresh grouper, snapper, mahi-mahi or haddock fillets
- 8-12 flour tortillas, soft
- 1 head shredded lettuce
- marinade
- 2 tablespoons olive oil
- 2 tablespoons garlic, minced
- 1 teaspoon cumin
- 1 teaspoon chili powder
- 2 tablespoons lime juice

Direction

- Combine fish fillets with marinade mixture and refrigerate for 1 hour. Grill fillets on a hot grill. Chop cooked fillets into bite-sized pieces. Fill tortilla with shredded lettuce, fish pieces, and Mango/Avocado Salsa.
- Mango/Avocado Salsa
- 2 mangos, diced medium
- 1 avocado, diced medium
- 1/4 cup red onion, diced
- 1 tablespoon jalapeno pepper, minced
- 2 tablespoons cilantro, chopped
- 1 tablespoon lime juice
- 1 tablespoon olive oil
- Salt and pepper to taste
- Preparation
- Combine all ingredients; mix well and refrigerate until ready to use.

120. Grilled Halibut Recipe

Serving: 1 | Prep: | Cook: 8mins | Ready in:

Ingredients

- Fresh if possible halibut steak
- fresh lemon
- salt and pepper
- asparagus
- vegetable Supreme
- Mayo Best Foods or Hellmans
- olive oil

Direction

- Wash steaks, pat dry.
- Liberally coat with olive oil and salt and pepper to taste.
- Grill on medium high on gas grill over open flame about 4-5 minutes per side.
- Cook asparagus to your taste.
- Spread mayo on spears and top with sprinkling of Vegetable Supreme

121. Grilled Halibut With Eggplant And Baby Bok Choy And Korean Barbecue Sauce Recipe

Serving: 4 | Prep: | Cook: 30mins | Ready in:

Ingredients

- 4 tablespoons olive oil or vegetable oil, divided
- 2 garlic cloves, minced
- 1 1/2 teaspoons minced serrano chile with seeds (they add a great flavor and zip
- 1/3 cup soy sauce
- 1/4 cup (packed) dark brown sugar
- 3 tablespoons unseasoned rice vinegar
- 3 tablespoons water
- 1 tablespoon Asian sesame oil
- ~~~~
- 8 baby bok choy, halved lengthwise
- 4 medium-size Japanese eggplants, trimmed, halved lengthwise
- 4 6- to 7-ounce halibut fillets (each about 1 inch thick)
- 2 green onions, thinly sliced

Direction

- Heat 1 tablespoon olive oil in heavy small saucepan over medium heat.
- Add garlic and chili; sauté until fragrant and light golden, about 3 minutes.
- Add soy sauce, brown sugar, vinegar, and 3 tablespoons water and bring to boil, stirring until sugar dissolves.
- Reduce heat to medium and simmer until mixture is reduced to 3/4 cup, about 5 minutes (sauce will be thin).
- Remove barbecue sauce from heat; whisk in sesame oil.
- Transfer 1/4 cup barbecue sauce to small bowl and reserve for serving.
- **You can make the sauce up to 24 hours early.
- ~~~~
- Prepare grill (medium heat).
- Combine bok choy and eggplant halves in large bowl. Drizzle 2 tablespoons olive oil over and toss to coat. Sprinkle with salt and pepper.
- Brush fish with remaining 1 tablespoon olive oil; sprinkle with salt and pepper.
- Grill vegetables and fish until vegetables are tender and slightly charred and fish is just opaque in center, turning occasionally and brushing with sauce, about 10 minutes total for vegetables and 7 minutes total for fish.
- Transfer vegetables and fish to plates; sprinkle with green onions.
- Drizzle with reserved sauce and serve.

122. Grilled Halibut With Pineapple Salsa Recipe

Serving: 4 | Prep: | Cook: 20mins | Ready in:

Ingredients

- 1/2 pineapple peeled cored and chopped
- 1 granny smith apple cored and grated
- 1 teaspoon grated fresh ginger
- 1/2 lemon juice and zest
- 1 teaspoon salt
- 1 teaspoon hot chili flakes
- 4 halibut steaks
- 1 tablespoon vanilla oil
- 1 tablespoon grated fresh ginger
- 1/2 lemon zest only
- 1/2 teaspoon hot chili flakes
- 1 tablespoon minced fresh thyme

Direction

- Combine pineapple, apple, ginger, lemon juice, zest, salt and hot chili flakes.
- Stir well then cover and let stand to allow the flavors to blend.
- Lightly oil fish then sprinkle with ginger, lemon zest, hot chili flakes and thyme.
- Heat grill to high and grill fish turning once.
- Serve with pineapple compote on the side.

123. Grilled Jack Daniels Salmon Recipe

Serving: 4 | Prep: | Cook: 15mins | Ready in:

Ingredients

- 2 salmon fillets (enough for 3 to 4 servings. 6-8 oz each)
- 1/2 c Jack Daniels Whiskey
- 1/2 c brown sugar
- 1/4 c soy sauce
- 2 tablespoons honey
- 1/2 tsp ground ginger
- salt & pepper, to taste
- aluminum foil

Direction

- Preheat grill.
- Meanwhile, in a small saucepan combine Jack Daniels, brown sugar, soy sauce, honey, & ginger.
- Bring to boiling.
- Lower heat to medium setting, continually stirring mixture until liquid is thickened and caramelized.
- Remove from heat. Salt and pepper the salmon fillets.
- Create a foil platter for your Salmon to grill upon by folding all 4 edges of the foil such that it creates a 1/2" lip around the platter.
- Place fillets skin side down on foil and grill on a low heat setting. Brush Jack sauce on fillets.
- Cook for about 7 minutes.
- Flip the Salmon fillets; the skin should stick to the foil platter.
- Continue to baste fillets with the caramelized Jack sauce about every 3 minutes until fillets are cooked thoroughly.
- (About 15 minutes or until Salmon has a light pink color in the middle.)
- Serve immediately

124. Grilled King Salmon Roasted Fennel And Goat Cheese Feta Hash Lemon Cucumber Vinaigrette Recipe

Serving: 6 | Prep: | Cook: 40mins | Ready in:

Ingredients

- #
- roasted fennel & goat cheese Hash
- Ingredients:
- 1 Large bulb of fennel
- 1 large red pepper, roasted and peeled
- 1 cup sliced onions (red, Spanish, shallots or cipollini can be used)
- 3 Lbs. potatoes (redskin, Yukon gold or any variety can be used)
- 3 T. fresh oregano
- Blended oil
- salt & pepper
- 1/2 cup Vermont goat cheese feta
- Lemon cucumber Vinaigrette
- Ingredients:
- 1 cup minced seedless cucumber
- 3 T. chopped shallots
- 1 T. chopped fresh garlic
- 3 T. capers
- 1/4 cup fresh lemon juice
- 2 cups blended oil
- salt and pepper

Direction

- Directions Roasted Fennel & Goat Cheese Hash
- Ingredients:
- Cut the leaves off of the fennel bulb and reserve. Cut the bulb in half and separate. Place the fennel on a sheet pan. Coat the fennel in oil and lightly salt and pepper. Place the sheet pan in a preheated 400-degree oven. Roast the fennel until it is soft. When the fennel is cool, slice and reserve.

- Roast the red peppers using the above procedure. When the peppers are soft, remove them from the pan into a bowl and cover with plastic wrap for 15-20 minutes. This process will allow the pepper skin to steam off. When the peppers are ready, remove the plastic and peel the skins off, chop the peppers and reserve.
- Sauté the onions until translucent, reserve.
- In a large mixing bowl, toss the fennel, peppers, potatoes and onions together. Chop the fresh oregano and add to the mixture. This mixture can be made a day ahead of time and keep in the refrigerator for up to 3 days.
- When you reheat the hash, add the goat cheese at the last minute so it does not melt all the way. Adjust the seasoning with salt and pepper.
- Procedure
- Mince the cucumbers and set aside.
- In a food processor fitted with a metal blade, place the shallots, garlic and capers. Pulse quickly for a few seconds.
- Add the lemon juice and process. Slowly add the oil. Remove the mixture to a small mixing bowl.
- Add the cucumbers and adjust the seasoning with salt and pepper.
- To Serve
- Grill or sauté a piece of salmon (you may substitute any fish, but the richness of the salmon holds up well with the stronger flavors in the hash and vinaigrette).
- Heat a skillet over medium-high heat and add 1 T. of oil. When the oil is hot. Add the hash mixture, toss frequently until the mix is hot, turn the heat off and add the feta cheese.
- Place a mound of hash in the center of the plate. Place the Salmon on top of the hash.
- Surround the hash with some cucumber vinaigrette.
- Garnish the Salmon with some micro greens or some herb salad.

125. Grilled Lemon Garlic Halibut Steaks Recipe

Serving: 4 | Prep: | Cook: 10mins | Ready in:

Ingredients

- 1/4 cup lemon juice
- 1 tablespoon vegetable oil
- 1/4 teaspoon salt
- 1/4 teaspoon pepper
- 2 cloves garlic, finely chopped
- 4 halibut or tuna steaks, about 1 inch thick (about 2 pounds)
- 1/4 cup chopped fresh parsley
- 1 tablespoon grated lemon peel

Direction

- Brush grill rack with vegetable oil.
- Heat coals or gas grill for direct heat.
- In shallow glass or plastic dish or resealable food-storage plastic bag, mix lemon juice, 1 tablespoon oil, the salt, pepper and garlic. Add fish; turn several times to coat with marinade.
- Cover dish or seal bag and refrigerate 10 minutes.
- Remove fish from marinade; reserve marinade.
- Cover and grill fish 4 to 6 inches from medium heat 10 to 15 minutes, turning once and brushing with marinade, until fish flakes easily with fork.
- Discard any remaining marinade.
- Sprinkle fish with parsley and lemon peel.

126. Grilled Mahi Mahi Ceviche Style Recipe

Serving: 4 | Prep: | Cook: 8mins | Ready in:

Ingredients

- 4 skinless mahi-mahi filets, approximately 2 pounds

- 2 tsp kosher salt
- 1/2 diced red onion
- 1/4 cup freshly squeezed lime juice
- 1/4 cup of orange juice
- 1 tbs minced jalapeno
- 1/4 cup dark brown sugar, packed
- 1/4 cup tequila
- 1 tbs olive oil
- 1/4 cup freshly chopped cilantro leaves

Direction

- Rub the fillets with kosher salt and set aside in a non-reactive bowl
- Combine onion, lime juice, orange juice, jalapeno, sugar, cilantro leaves and tequila, I just put it all in the blender.
- Put filets and mixture into zip lock bag marinade for 2 hours in refrigerator.
- Remove the fillets from the marinade and set it aside.
- Transfer remaining marinade to a saucepan and heat until it is reduced to about 3/4 cup. You may want to start this while fish is reaching room temperature.
- Pat the fillets dry with paper towels and lightly coat with the olive oil.
- Heat grill to med-high and place the fillets over direct heat until they are just cooked through-opaque at the center but still moist, approximately 3-4 mins per side.
- Serve with marinade sauce and extra cilantro on top.
- ENJOY

127. Grilled Red Snapper With Avocado Papaya Salsa Diabetic Friendly Recipe

Serving: 4 | Prep: | Cook: 10mins | Ready in:

Ingredients

- Ingredients:
- 1 tsp. ground coriander
- 1 tsp. paprika
- ¾ tsp. salt
- ¼ tsp. ground red pepper
- 1 Tbs. olive oil
- 4 skinless red snapper or halibut fish fillets (5 to 7oz each)
- ½ cup diced ripe avocado
- 2 Tbs. cilantro chopped
- 1 Tbs. fresh lime juice
- 4 Lime wedges

Direction

- 1) Prepare grill for direct grilling. Combine coriander, paprika, salt and red pepper in a small bowl or cup; mix well.
- 2) Brush oil over fish. Sprinkle 2 ½ tsp. Spice mixture over fish fillets; set aside remaining spice mixture. Place fish skin side down on oiled grid over medium-hot heat. Grill 5 minutes per side or until fish is opaque.
- 3) Meanwhile, combine avocado, papaya, cilantro, lime juice and reserved spice mixture in a medium bowl; mix well. Serve fish with salsa and garnish with lime wedges. Makes 4 servings.
- Nutritional Values: Calories per serving: 221, Fat 9g, Carbohydrate 5g, Cholesterol 51mg, Sodium 559mg
- Note: This is a Diabetic Friendly recipe.

128. Grilled Salmon Fillet With Honey Mustard Sauce Recipe

Serving: 4 | Prep: | Cook: 10mins | Ready in:

Ingredients

- 1/4 cup Dijon mustard
- 2 tablespoons whole-grain mustard
- 3 tablespoons honey
- 2 tablespoons prepared horseradish, drained
- 2 tablespoons finely chopped fresh mint leaves
- kosher salt and freshly ground black pepper

- 2 pound fillet salmon, skin on
- 2 tablespoons canola oil
- 1 bunch watercress, coarsely chopped
- 1 small red onion, halved and thinly sliced
- 2 tablespoons aged sherry vinegar
- 2 tablespoons extra-virgin olive oil

Direction

- Whisk together the mustards, honey, horseradish, mint and 1/4 teaspoon of salt and 1/4 teaspoon of pepper in a small bowl. Let sit for at least 15 minutes before using. Can be made 1 day in advance and refrigerated but do not add the mint until just before using. Bring to room temperature before using.
- Heat the grill to high.
- Brush the salmon with the oil and season with salt and pepper. Place the salmon on the grill, skin side down, and grill until golden brown and slightly charred, about 3 minutes.
- While the salmon is cooking, place the watercress and onion in a medium bowl, add the vinegar and oil and salt and pepper and toss to combine. Transfer the salad to a platter, top with the salmon fillet and drizzle each fillet with the mustard sauce.

129. Grilled Salmon Fillets Recipe

Serving: 2 | Prep: | Cook: 15mins | Ready in:

Ingredients

- 1 pound fresh salmon fillets (wild salmon preferred)
- 2 cloves minced garlic
- 1 T olive oil
- 1/4 c chopped fresh parsley
- salt/pepper

Direction

- Heat grill.
- Prepare salmon fillets by placing them on a sheet of aluminum foil. Salt liberally, then add pepper, garlic, olive oil and parsley.
- Once the grill reaches a medium-high heat, place foil containing salmon onto grill.
- Close lid.
- Keep a close watch on the salmon.
- Depending on the thickness, it should be done in 10-15 minutes.
- Test for doneness with a fork.
- If fish flakes easily, it is done.
- Can cook on an indoor grill 5-7 minutes or 5-7 minutes per side, depending on the type of grill used.

130. Grilled Salmon With Lime Butter Sauce Recipe

Serving: 6 | Prep: | Cook: 15mins | Ready in:

Ingredients

- 6 (6-oz) pieces center-cut salmon fillet (about 1 inch thick) with skin
- 1 1/2 teaspoons finely grated fresh lime zest
- ****
- NOTE: It takes only 5 minutes to make this fantastic Lime butter Sauce. Once you see how versatile it is – it works perfectly with the grilled salmon and the grilled corn on the menu – you'll want to make it for a whole host of your summer favorites.
- **
- Lime butter Sauce: (You'll need 6 tablespoons for the salmon - reserve the rest for the Grilled corn with herbs or some other lucky dish.)
- 1 large garlic clove, chopped
- 1/4 cup fresh lime juice
- 1 teaspoon salt
- 1/2 teaspoon black pepper
- 1 stick (1/2 cup) unsalted butter, melted

Direction

- Lime Butter Sauce:

- Purée garlic with lime juice, salt, and pepper in a blender until smooth.
- With motor running, add melted butter and blend until emulsified, about 30 seconds.
- Reserve 6 tablespoons for salmon.
- Lime Butter Sauce Note: Lime butter sauce can be made 1 day ahead and chilled, covered. Stir before using.
- Makes about 3/4 cup.
- ****
- Prepare grill for cooking over medium-hot charcoal (moderate heat for gas).
- Season salmon all over with salt and pepper, then grill, flesh sides down, on lightly oiled grill rack (covered only if using gas grill) for 4 minutes.
- Turn fillets over and grill (covered only if using gas grill) until just cooked through, 4 to 6 minutes more.
- Sprinkle fillets with zest and top each with 1 tablespoon prepared Lime Butter Sauce.
- ****
- STOVETOP INSTRUCTIONS:
- Salmon Note: If you aren't able to grill outdoors or don't care to, the salmon can be cooked in a hot well-seasoned large pan on the stovetop over moderately high heat. As follows -
- Heat large sauté pan over medium-high heat.
- When hot, add 1-2 tablespoons of olive oil and 1 tablespoon of unsalted butter. When the butter melts completely into the olive oil, add the salted and peppered salmon fillets, flesh side down.
- Watch the salmon closely. You do not want to overcook it.
- I would estimate 4-6 minutes per side. HOWEVER, I don't time the process as much as I watch the "cook line" of the salmon. In that I mean, you can see the salmon turning a lighter pink as it cooks and it will move up the fillet from the pan surface. Watch the center sides where the thickness is.
- As the cook line gets almost half way up the center thickness of the fillet, flip the fillet into the skin side. Cook another 4 minutes or until the cook line gets close to the done line above.
- What you want: To leave about 1/8 inch of uncooked salmon in the very center of the thickness part of the fillet. Remove from pan and place on serving platter.
- **The salmon will continue to cook after it is removed from the heat. But the perfectly cooked salmon fillet here is still a tiny bit on the just-barely-cooked side in the dead center. That way it remains moist and flaky and perfect throughout
- Sprinkle fillets with zest and top each with 1 tablespoon lime butter sauce.

131. Grilled Salmon With Nectarine Red Onion Relish Recipe

Serving: 4 | Prep: | Cook: 12mins | Ready in:

Ingredients

- 2 1/2 cups coarsely chopped nectarines (about 3 medium)
- 1 cup coarsley chopped red bell pepper
- 1 cup coarsely chopped red onion
- 1/4 cup thinly sliced fresh basil
- 1/4 cup white wine vinegar
- 1/2 tps. grated orange peel
- 1/4 cup fresh orange juice
- 2 TBSP. minced seeded jalapeno pepper
- 2 TBSP. fresh lime juice
- 2 tps. sugar
- 2 garlic cloves minced
- 1/4 tps. salt, divded
- 1/2 tps. freshly groun pepper
- 4 (6-ounce) fillets
- 1/2

Direction

- 1. Combine first 11 ingredients and 1/8 tsp. salt in a medium bowl, and stir well. Let nectarine mixture stand 2 hours.

- 2. Sprinkle pepper and 1/8 teaspoon salt over salmon fillets. Prepare grill. Place fillets on a grill rack coated with cooking spray, and grill 5-6 minutes on each side or until fish flakes easily when tested with a fork. Serve immediately with nectarine-red onion relish.
- 3. Serving size: 1 fillet and 1 cup relish.

132. Grilled Sea Bass With Orange And Red Onion Sauce And Citrus Couscous Recipe

Serving: 6 | Prep: | Cook: 50mins | Ready in:

Ingredients

- orange and red onion Sauce:
- 1½ Tbsp olive oil
- 1 lb red onions, cut into ¼-inch slices
- 2 cups freshly squeezed orange juice
- 2 Tbsp flat-leaf parsley, finely chopped
- Dash of Tabasco sauce
- Pinch of ground coriander
- ¼ tsp salt
- Freshly ground black pepper to taste
- Citrus Couscous:
- 3 cups light chicken stock
- Grated zest of 1 orange
- Grated zest of 1 lemon
- Grated zest of 1 lime
- ¼ tsp Chinese chile paste
- 2 Tbsp extra virgin olive oil
- 1½ cups instant couscous
- ½ tsp salt
- ¼ tsp freshly ground black pepper
- Grilled Sea Bass:
- 6 (4- to 5-ounce) skinless, boneless sea bass fillets, about 1-inch thick
- 1 Tbsp olive oil
- ½ lemon
- salt and freshly ground black pepper
- Sprigs of chervil

Direction

- Heat olive oil in a large skillet over medium-low heat.
- Add red onions and sauté, stirring occasionally, for about 10 minutes, or until the onions are softened but not browned.
- Add orange juice and bring mixture to a boil. Simmer until the liquid is reduced by half, about 10 minutes.
- Remove from heat and stir in parsley, Tabasco, coriander, salt, and pepper. Set aside.
- In a medium saucepan, combine stock, citrus zests, chile paste, and olive oil.
- Bring the mixture just to a boil over medium heat, and then immediately stir in couscous.
- Remove from heat, cover pan, and let stand until the couscous is tender, about 10 minutes.
- When all of the liquid has been absorbed, fluff the couscous with a fork and add salt and pepper.
- Brush sea bass fillets on all sides with olive oil.
- Preheat a grill or broiler to medium-high.
- Season fillets with salt and pepper and grill them for about 3 minutes on each side, or until done through and opaque.
- During the last minute of cooking, squeeze a little lemon juice over each fillet.
- To plate, put a mound of couscous on each of 6 heated dinner plates and place a grilled fillet on top.
- Drizzle the onion sauce around the edge of the plates and garnish with a few sprigs of chervil.

133. Grilled Swordfish Recipe

Serving: 6 | Prep: | Cook: 15mins | Ready in:

Ingredients

- 1 Tbl EVOO
- 1/2 C finely chopped shallots
- 1 Tbl finely chopped thyme (1/2 the amount if dried)
- 1/2 tsp sugar
- 1/2 tsp lemon peel

- 2 Tbl Dijon mustard
- 2 Tbl white wine or water
- 2 Lb swordfish, cut into 6 serving size pieces

Direction

- Heat Grill or broiler
- In a small non-stick skillet, heat oil over medium heat until hot
- Add shallots; cook and stir about 3 minutes or until tender
- Remove from heat and stir in thyme, sugar, lemon peel, mustard and wine or water until well blended
- Spread 1/2 the mixture on one side of swordfish
- Oil grill rack or spray broiler pan (or line a 15 x 10x 1 pan with foil)
- Grill or broil 4 to 6 inches from heat for about 6 to 7 minutes
- Turn fish and spread with remaining mixture
- Cook an additional 7 minutes or until fish slakes easily with a fork
- If broiling, mixture will be lightly browned
- 6 servings

134. Grilled Swordfish With Melon Salsa Recipe

Serving: 4 | Prep: | Cook: 15mins | Ready in:

Ingredients

- 2 pounds fresh, boneless swordfish steak about 1-inch thick-cut into 4 pieces
- 1 1/2 cups cantaloupe, peeled and diced
- 1 1/2 cups honeydew, peeled and diced
- 1 1/2 cups mango, peeled and diced
- 1/2 cup greenbell pepper, chopped fine
- 1/2 cup red pepper, chopped fine
- 1/3 cup red onion, chopped fine
- 4 ounces green chilies, diced
- 2 tbsps. fresh cilantro, chopped
- 1 clove garlic, minced or chopped fine
- 3 tbsps. fresh lime juice- sqoeezed from lime
- 1 tbsp. white wine vinegar
- 1 tsp. canoal oil 1/2 tsp. ground cumin
- salt and pepper to taste

Direction

- 1. Slice cantaloupe, honeydew and mango, removing the fruit so it can be diced into 1/4 inch cubes. Chop the green pepper, red pepper, and red onion into fine pieces. If chilies are not diced or seeded, remove the seeds and cut into fine pieces. Chop fresh cilantro and garlic into small pieces. Place those ingredients in a small mixing bowl and toss well.
- 2. In a separate bowl, squeeze 3 TBSPS. from one lime and mix with vinegar, oil, and ground cumin. Pour contents into the fruit mixture, mixing all together. Cover and refrigerate for several hours to allow flavors to combine.
- 3. Preheat grill on medium heat for 3-4 minutes. Brush grill surface with cooking oil.
- 4. Grill fish for about 4 to 7 minutes on each side or until steaks are firm to the touch, but still moist, tender, and slightly opaque on the inside at the thickest point.

135. Grilled Tandoori Fish And Chips Recipe

Serving: 4 | Prep: | Cook: 8mins | Ready in:

Ingredients

- Fish:
- 1-1/2 c plain yogurt
- 2 tsp ea. garlic paste,grated fresh ginger,paprika
- 1 tsp ea. currt powder,red chili powder,ground cumin
- 1/2 tsp salt
- 4 (6oz) 3/4" thick tilapia,snaper or mahimahi fillets

- Chips:
- 2 (8oz) gearnet yams or sweet potatoes,halved lengthwise,cut in 3/4" wedges
- 2 Tbs ghee or unsalted butter,melted
- 1 tsp garam masala
- 1/4 tsp ea coarse sea salt and freshly ground black pepper
- olive oil for brushing

Direction

- In large bowl, whisk together yogurt, ginger, garlic paste, paprika, curry powder, chili, cumin powder and salt. Remove 1 cup of mixture and reserve for serving.
- Place fillets in shallow dish and brush with remaining yogurt mixture to coat completely. Cover, refrigerate 1 hour.
- Chips: Place yam wedges, skin-side down, on large microwave-safe plate; cover with vented plastic wrap. Microwave on high 3-1/2 to 4 mins or till almost tender; let cool.
- Heat outdoor grill on med-high heat. Mix ghee, garam masala, salt and pepper in large bowl; add yam wedges and gently toss to coat.
- Remove fillets from marinade; wipe off excess. Brush the cooking grates with oil. Lightly brush fillets with oil. Grill fillets and yams (keeping grill closed as much as possible) until fish is opaque and still moist and yams lightly charred, 6 to 8 mins, carefully turning fillets once when fish releases easily from grill pan and turning yam wedges as they brown. Serve with remaining yogurt mixture.

136. Grilled Teriyaki Mahi Mahi With Mango Salsa Recipe

Serving: 4 | Prep: | Cook: 10mins | Ready in:

Ingredients

- salsa recipe
- 1/4 cup finely chopped red onion
- 1 tablespoon vegetable oil
- 1 tablespoon fresh lime juice
- 1 tablespoon finely chopped fresh mint
- 1 teaspoon minced jalapeno pepper, with seeds
- 1/4 teaspoon kosher salt
- marinade recipe
- 1/4 cup soy sauce (La Choy is wheat free)
- 1/4 cup sweet sake
- 1 tablespoon vegetable oil
- 1 tablespoon light brown sugar
- 1 teaspoon grated fresh ginger
- 1 teaspoon minced garlic
- 4 mahi mahi fillets, about 6 oz. each and 1 inch thick
- vegetable oil

Direction

- For the salsa: Peel the mango and cut into 1/4 inch diced pieces.
- Put mango pieces in a small bowl with the remaining salsa ingredients; stir to combine.
- Cover bowl with saran wrap and refrigerate until ready to serve.
- For the marinade: In a small bowl, whisk together the soy sauce, sweet sake, vegetable oil, light brown sugar, fresh ginger, and minced garlic; set aside.
- Place the mahi-mahi fillets in a large zip-lock plastic bag.
- Pour marinade into bag; press the air out of the bag and seal tightly.
- Turn/shake the bag to coat fillets with marinade.
- Refrigerate for 20-30 minutes.
- Take fillets out of bag and throw away marinade.
- Brush or spray both sides of fillets with vegetable oil.
- Grill over high heat until fish is opaque throughout, 8 to 10 minutes, turning once halfway through grilling time.
- Serve warm with salsa.

137. Grilled Teriyaki Tuna Recipe

Serving: 4 | Prep: | Cook: | Ready in:

Ingredients

- 4 (4 oz) yellowfin tuna filets
- 1 cup of teriyaki sauce
- 2 tbsp garlic, minced
- 3/4 cup olive oil
- 1 tsp ground black pepper

Direction

- Combine the teriyaki sauce, oil, pepper and garlic. Place that mixture, along with the tuna fillets, in a large resealable plastic bag. Remove as much air as possible, and seal the bag. To make sure the tuna fillets are well coated, shake the mixture well. Place the bag in the refrigerator and marinate for 30 minutes. Then, preheat your outdoor grill at a high heat, and lightly oil the grate. Take out the tuna from the marinade, and put on the grill. Grill for 3-5 minutes on each side (for rare tuna), 5-8 minutes per side (for medium) and 8-10 minutes per side (for well done).
- NOTE: Cooking times will depend on the thickness of the tuna fillets, and the heat of your grill. To check the doneness, make a cut with a knife and check the color in the middle of the filet.

138. Grilled Teriyaki Tuna Wraps Recipe

Serving: 8 | Prep: | Cook: 8mins | Ready in:

Ingredients

- 3 -> 8 ounce, 1 inch thick fresh tuna steaks
- 1/3 cup soy sauce (recommend Low sodium)
- 2 cloves garlic, minced.
- 1-1/2 tspn packed brown sugar
- 1-1/2 tspn finely shredded or grated ginger
- 1 Tbsp light olive oil
- 3/4 cup fat free sour cream
- 3/4 bottle honey mustard salad dressing
- 2 cups lightly packed arugula leaves
- 1 large red onion, sliced (~ 1 cup)
- 1 medium tomato, chopped
- 8 10 inch flour tortillas

Direction

- (Marinade) In a small bowl, stir together soy sauce, garlic, sugar, and ginger.
- Place fish in a resealable plastic bag, pour in marinade, seal and set in a shallow dish in the refrigerator.
- Marinate for 1 to 2 hours turning bag occasionally. Drain and discard marinade just prior to grilling the tuna.
- Grilling: a) For a charcoal grill, grill the fish on a greased rack of an uncovered grill over medium coals to 8 to 12 minutes (fish should flake easily... don't overcook or it will get tough) turning once. b) For a gas grill, preheat the grill, reduce heat to medium, place fish on grease grill rack, cover and grill as above.
- After grilling the tuna, cut it into 1/2 inch chunks.
- Brush both side of tortillas lightly with olive oil and grill for 30 to 45 seconds or until warm.
- In a medium bowl, stir together the sour cream and salad dressing.
- For each wrap, spread 3 Tbsp of the sour cream mixture on the tortilla.
- Place some tuna near an edge of the tortilla
- Top with arugula, onion, and tomato.
- Fold edge over filling, fold in the sides and roll up

139. HADDOCK WITH TOMATO AND ONION SALSA Recipe

Serving: 4 | Prep: | Cook: 6mins | Ready in:

Ingredients

- 1 red onion halved and thinly sliced
- 4 tomatoes, halved with cores removed
- 1 tsp crushed chili flakes
- 1 tsp grated fresh ginger
- 1 tsp sugar
- 1 tbsp tomato paste
- 1 tbsp balsamic vinegar
- 3 tbsp olive oil'divided
- 4 haddock fillets

Direction

- Separate onion slices into shreds and put into a bowl.
- Thinly slice tomatoes and add to onions.
- Sprinkle with chili flakes, ginger and sugar.
- Stir in tomato paste and vinegar.
- Stir in 2 tbsp of olive oil.
- Set aside.
- Preheat broiler to high, lightly grease broiler pan.
- Put on Haddock, skin side up, and brush with remaining oil.
- Cook 3 minutes.
- Turn fish and cook 3 minutes more or until cooked through.
- Divide salsa among 4 plates.
- Lay haddock on top.
- Serve.

140. Haddock Filets In Wine Sauce Recipe

Serving: 6 | Prep: | Cook: 25mins | Ready in:

Ingredients

- 1 1/2 pounds skinless haddock filets, cut into serving pieces
- 1 green onion, thinly sliced
- 1/2 cup fresh mushrooms, thinly sliced (I use more)
- 2 large ripe tomatoes, seeded and coarsely chopped
- 1 cup white wine
- 1 teaspoon curry powder
- 1 cup light cream
- 1 teaspoon salt, or to taste
- 1/4 teaspoon ground white pepper
- 1/2 cup dry breadcrumbs
- 1/2 cup sharp cheddar cheese, shredded
- 2 tablespoons butter, melted
- lemon wedges

Direction

- Arrange fish filets in a greased 13x9 inch baking dish.
- Sprinkle fish with green onion, mushrooms and tomato.
- Combine wine and curry powder. Pour over filets.
- Bake at 325 degrees for 15 to 20 minutes or until fish filets flake easily.
- Remove from oven and carefully lift out fish filets and set aside.
- In saucepan, heat cream. Add pan juices to saucepan. Add salt and pepper. Heat just to a boil.
- Return filets to baking pan.
- Pour cream mixture over.
- Combine crumbs and cheese. Sprinkle over filets.
- Drizzle with melted butter.
- Broil until crumbs and cheese are golden brown.
- Serve with lemon wedges.

141. Haddock Fish Fillets With Wine Sauce Dated 1943 Recipe

Serving: 2 | Prep: | Cook: 30mins | Ready in:

Ingredients

- 2 tablespoons minced onion
- 1 tablespoon oil
- 2 tablespoons flour
- 1-1/2 teaspoons salt
- 1/8 teaspoon pepper
- 1/2 cup cream
- 1/2 cup sauterne wine
- 1 pound fresh haddock fillets
- 1 tablespoon chopped fresh parsley

Direction

- Sauté onion in hot oil in a heavy enameled pan or double boiler until tender.
- Stir in the flour, salt, and pepper blending well.
- Add milk stirring constantly and cook until thick.
- When thickened remove and very gradually stir in the wine.
- Put the fish in a baking pan and sprinkle with salt.
- Pour sauce over fish.
- Bake at 350 for thirty minutes basting often.
- Sprinkle with parsley and serve.

142. Halibut Alla Diavola With Lemon Parsley Couscous Recipe

Serving: 4 | Prep: | Cook: 35mins | Ready in:

Ingredients

- halibut - tomato sauce
- 4 halibut or sea bass Filets (4 oz each)
- salt and pepper
- 3 T all-purpose flour
- 1 med onion, sliced
- 1/2 c pitted kalamata olives, halved
- 2 garlic cloves, thinly sliced
- 4 c quartered roma tomatoes
- 2 t red pepper flakes
- 1 t Dijon mustard
- 1 c dry white wine
- 1/4 c brandy
- lemon PARSLEY couscous
- 1 3/4 c chicken broth
- 1/4 c fresh lemon juice
- 1 1/2 c plain dry couscous
- 1 T olive oil
- 2 T chopped fresh parsley
- 1 t lemon zest
- salt to taste
- lemon wedges for serving

Direction

- HALIBUT - TOMATO SAUCE
- Season fish with salt and pepper, then dredge one side of filets in flour
- Sauté fish, floured side down, in oil in a large sauté pan over medium high heat, until golden brown, 3 minutes
- Transfer filets to a plate, reduce heat to medium
- Add onion, olives and garlic, sauté 2 minutes
- Stir in tomatoes, pepper flakes, and mustard.
- Deglaze with white wine and brandy
- Reduce heat to medium-low and simmer until thickened, 15 minutes
- Lightly mash tomatoes with a spoon to break them up
- Arrange filets on top of tomato mixture, browned side up
- Cover with a tight-fitting lid and simmer until fish flakes easily when tested with a fork, 5-7 minutes
- LEMON-PARSLEY COUSCOUS
- Meanwhile
- Bring chicken broth, lemon juice and olive oil to a boil
- Remove from heat
- Stir in couscous, parsley and zest
- Cover and let stand 5 minutes
- Fluff with a fork, then season with salt

143. Halibut Bake Recipe

Serving: 6 | Prep: | Cook: | Ready in:

Ingredients

- 2 pounds halibut fillets, skinless
- 3/4 cup sour cream
- 3/4 cup mayonnaise
- 3/4 cup salsa
- 1/4 cup melted butter
- 1 tbsp garlic oil
- lemon pepper, to taste

Direction

- Preheat oven to 350 degrees F.
- Pour the butter into a baking dish and place the halibut fillets in the dish. Then, season with the lemon pepper.
- Combine the sour cream, mayonnaise, salsa, and garlic oil in a bowl, then spoon onto the halibut fillets.
- Bake for 30 minutes (fish should easily flake with a fork).

144. Halibut Monterey Recipe

Serving: 4 | Prep: | Cook: 20mins | Ready in:

Ingredients

- Ingredients:
- 2 pounds boneless, skinless halibut fillets, cut into 4 equal portions
- Stuffing:
- 3/4 cup crab meat or substitute shrimp
- 1/2 cup shredded pepperjack cheese
- 2 thinly sliced green onions
- 2 tablespoons water chestnuts, cut into thin strips
- 2 tablespoons bacon, fried crisp and finely chopped
- 2 tablespoons roasted red peppers, chopped
- 2 tablespoons mayonnaise
- 1 tablespoon lemon juice

Direction

- Combine all of the stuffing ingredients and mix thoroughly. Set aside.
- Using a thin sharp knife, cut a deep pocket in the top or side of each halibut portion. Be careful not to cut closer than 1/2-inch from either edge.
- Preheat oven to 400 degrees.
- Using a teaspoon and the tip of your finger, gently stuff each portion with the crab mixture, taking care not to tear the pocket.
- Place stuffed fillet portions on lightly greased baking sheet and bake in preheated oven for 18-20 minutes.

145. Halibut Steaks Recipe

Serving: 4 | Prep: | Cook: 14mins | Ready in:

Ingredients

- 1/2 cup soy sauce
- 1/4 cup packed brown sugar
- 2 garlic cloves, minced
- 1/8 tps. pepper
- Dash hot pepper sauce
- pinch dried oregano
- pinch dried basil
- 4 halibut steaks (6 ounces each)
- 1/2 cup chopped onion
- 4 lemon slices
- 4 tps. butter

Direction

- 1. In a small bowl, combine the first seven ingredients
- 2. Place each halibut steak on a double thickness of heavy-duty foil (about 18x 12 inches) top with soy sauce mixture, onion, lemon, and butter. Fold foil around fish and seal tightly.

- 3. Grill, covered, over medium heat for 10 to 14 minutes or until fish flakes easily with a fork.

146. Halibut Steaks With Moroccan Spiced Oil Recipe

Serving: 4 | Prep: | Cook: 20mins | Ready in:

Ingredients

- 1 teaspoon coriander seeds
- 1 teaspoon cumin seeds
- 1/2 teaspoon fennel seeds
- 1/8 teaspoon crushed red pepper
- 2-1/2 tablespoons extra virgin olive oil
- 4 halibut steaks
- 1/4 teaspoon salt
- 1/2 teaspoon freshly ground black pepper

Direction

- In a small skillet toast coriander, cumin and fennel seeds over moderate heat 3 minutes.
- Shake skillet often then transfer spices and red pepper to a spice grinder and grind to a powder.
- Return spices to skillet and add 2 tablespoons olive oil and cook over low heat just until warmed.
- Pour oil through a very fine strainer or a tea strainer and keep warm.
- In large non-stick skillet heat remaining oil until shimmering.
- Season fish with salt and pepper and cook over moderately high for 5 minutes.
- Turn and cook the other side until browned and the fish is just cooked through about 3 minutes.
- Transfer fish to warmed plates then drizzle with spiced oil and serve.

147. Halibut With Grilled Pineapple And Raisin Salsa Recipe

Serving: 6 | Prep: | Cook: 10mins | Ready in:

Ingredients

- halibut With Grilled pineapple and raisin salsa
- 1/2 cup raisins
- 1/2 cup dark rum
- 1 fresh pineapple trimmed cored and sliced
- vegetable oil as needed
- 2 chipotle peppers canned in adobo sauce rinsed seeded and finely diced
- juice of 1 lime
- Zest of 1/2 orange
- juice of 1/2 orange
- 1/4 cup extra virgin olive oil
- 1 green onion sliced
- 2 tablespoons finely chopped roasted red pepper
- 2 tablespoons finely chopped cilantro
- 1 teaspoon sea salt
- 6 halibut steaks
- 1 tablespoon lemon pepper seasoning

Direction

- Plump raisins in rum for 30 minutes then drain well. Heat grill to medium high. Brush pineapple with oil then grill until lightly caramelized on both sides. Cool slightly and cut into 1/2-inch pieces and place in mixing bowl.
- In separate bowl combine chipotles, lime juice, zest and orange juice. Whisk in olive oil vigorously. Pour over pineapple chunks then fold in green onions, red peppers, cilantro and raisins. Season with sea salt then set aside. Brush halibut with oil then grill 5 minute on each side turning only once. Season with lemon pepper and serve with salsa.

148. Halibut With Mango Salsa Recipe

Serving: 4 | Prep: | Cook: 10mins | Ready in:

Ingredients

- 1 mango, diced
- 1/2 large red bell pepper, diced
- 1/4 cup diced red onion
- 3 tbsp finely chopped cilantro
- 2 tbsp lime juice
- 2 tbsp extra-virgin olive oil
- ½ -1 tsp. ground cumin
- 1/2 tsp. green Tabasco sauce
- 4 halibut fillets, about 6 ounces each
- salt to taste
- pepper to taste
- 1 tablespoon vegetable oil

Direction

- Combine mango, red pepper, and red onion in a bowl.
- In a separate bowl, combine lime juice, olive oil, cumin, and green Tabasco.
- Add to mango mix.
- Stir in cilantro and mix until well combined. Set aside.
- Season the halibut fillets with salt and pepper.
- In a large non-stick skillet, heat the oil over medium-high heat.
- Add the halibut fillets and sear the fillets for 4 to 6 minutes per side, depending on the thickness of the fillets.
- To serve, place fish on separate plates and top with salsa.

149. Halibut With Pasta In A Tomatoe Sauce John Style Recipe

Serving: 4 | Prep: | Cook: 40mins | Ready in:

Ingredients

- halibut (you can use chilean sea bass- or sea bass)
- 2 (10-ounce) halibut fillet,
- salt and freshly ground black pepper
- 1 tablespoon extra-virgin olive oil, plus 2 tablespoons
- 1 medium sized shallot, minced
- dash teaspoon red pepper flakes
- 3 tlsp flat-leaf Italian parsley, cleaned, stems removed, and chopped
- 2 garlic cloves, smashed and finely chopped
- 1/2 cup dry white wine
- 1 (28-ounce) can whole peeled tomatoes, crush with fingers
- 2 tlsp rinsed capers
- 1/2 cup pitted kalamata or green olives, smashed
- i med potatoe cut into small cubes and 2 slices of lemon cut in half
- I make it with pasta-(penne- or – rigatoni)

Direction

- Salt and pepper the halibut. Place 1 tablespoon of olive oil in a medium-sized, non-stick pan. When oil is shimmering, place the halibut, skin-side down, in pan. Cook on both sides for 2 minutes or to desirable color. Place halibut aside. In a medium-sized sauté pan over medium heat, add remaining 2 tablespoons of olive oil. Once it is hot, add the potatoes cook till almost done al dente, and then add the shallots, red pepper flakes, and parsley, and sauté for 2 minutes. Then add the garlic cloves, and cook another minute. Deglaze pan with 1/2 cup of the white wine and add tomatoes, capers, olives, Cook on low heat for 20 min- Start your pasta pot bring to a boil and cook pasta - as pasta is cooking add fish to the pan and sliced lemon, continue cooking till pasta is done add pasta to the pot and stir, serve hot.

150. Halibut And Capers Recipe

Serving: 4 | Prep: | Cook: 15mins | Ready in:

Ingredients

- 1 tablespoon olive oil
- 2 (8 ounce) halibut steaks
- 1/2 cup dry white wine
- 1 teaspoon garlic, chopped
- 1/4 cup butter
- salt and pepper to taste
- 3 tablespoons capers, with liquid

Direction

- Heat olive oil in a large skillet over medium high heat.
- Fry the halibut steaks on all sides until nicely browned.
- Remove from pan and set aside.
- Pour the wine into the pan and scrape up any browned bits.
- Let the wine reduce to almost nothing.
- Stir in garlic, butter and capers.
- Season with salt and pepper to taste.
- Allow sauce to simmer for a minute to meld flavors.
- Return steaks to pan and coat with sauce.
- Cook until fish is flaky when nudged with a fork.
- Serve fish immediately with sauce from the pan over it.

151. Halibut In Creamy Wine Sauce Recipe

Serving: 6 | Prep: | Cook: 180mins | Ready in:

Ingredients

- 2 (12oz. each) halibut steaks.
- 2 packages (10oz. each) frozen mixed vegetables, partially thawed
- 2 Tbs. flour
- 1 Tbs. sugar
- 1/4 tsp. salt
- 1/4 cup butter
- 1/3 cup white wine
- 2/3 cup half and half
- lemon wedges

Direction

- 1. Pat halibut steaks dry; set aside. Place 1 package vegetables in greased Crock-Pot. Combine flour, sugar, and salt.
- 2. In saucepan, melt butter; stir in flour mixture. When well blended, add wine and 1/2 and 1/2 and cook over medium heat until thickened, stirring constantly. Allow sauce to boil 1 minute while stirring.
- 3. Pour half the sauce over vegetables in Crock-Pot. Add half of halibut steaks and remaining package of vegetables. Pour remaining half of sauce over vegetables and top with last of halibut.
- 4. Cover and cook on high setting for 1 hour, then on low 2 hours. Transfer halibut to serving platter; garnish with lemon. Stir sauce and vegetables; serve separately in a vegetable dish.

152. Halibut On Fresh Polenta With Pepper Oil Recipe

Serving: 4 | Prep: | Cook: 10mins | Ready in:

Ingredients

- 1 red bell pepper, skin removed with a vegetable peeler,
- seeded, and cut into 1 inch pieces (about 1 cup)
- 3/4 tsp. kosher salt
- 2 tbsp. extra virgin olive oil
- 2-1/2 cups corn kernels (from 4 ears of corn)
- 2 tbsp. unsalted butter
- 1/4 tsp. freshly ground black pepper

- 4 small halibut steaks (4 oz. each and 3/4" thick)
- 1 tbsp. chopped fresh chives

Direction

- Put the red pepper pieces in a blender with 1/4 tsp. of the salt and the olive oil and process until smooth. Transfer to a microwavable bowl.
- Bring about 1-1/2 quarts salted water to a boil in a large skillet.
- Meanwhile, put the corn kernels in a blender and process until smooth. (You will have about 2 cups)
- Heat the butter in a saucepan, and add the corn puree along with the remaining 1/2 tsp. salt and the pepper. Bring to a boil and cook for about 30 seconds, or until the puree thickens. Set aside while you poach the fish.
- Drop the halibut steaks into the boiling water. Reduce the heat to low and cook the fish at a low boil for 2 to 3 minutes, depending on the thickness of the fish and your own taste preferences.
- Meanwhile, heat the pepper oil in a microwave oven for 1 minute. Divide the corn puree among the four plates. Lift the fish out of the water with a skimmer or fish spatula, pat it dry with paper towels, and place a steak on top of the polenta on each plate. Spoon on the hot pepper oil, sprinkle on the chives, and serve immediately.

153. Halibut With Cilantro Garlic Butter Recipe

Serving: 4 | Prep: | Cook: | Ready in:

Ingredients

- 4 (6 oz) halibut filets
- 1 lime, sliced into wedges
- 1 tbsp fresh lime juice
- 1/2 cup fresh cilantro, chopped
- 2 tbsp butter
- 1 tbsp olive oil
- 3 cloves garlic, roughly chopped
- salt and pepper (to taste)

Direction

- Preheat a grill at high heat. Squeeze the lime juice from wedges onto the fish fillets, and season with salt and pepper.
- Grill the fillets, on each side for around 5 minutes (fish should be browned able to be flaked with a fork). Remove and place on a warm serving plate.
- In a skillet, heat the oil over medium heat. Add the garlic and cook until fragrant, (approximately 2 minutes). Mix in butter, the left over lime juice and cilantro. Serve the filets with the cilantro butter sauce.

154. Halibut With Fennel Sun Dried Tomatoes And Olives Recipe

Serving: 4 | Prep: | Cook: 15mins | Ready in:

Ingredients

- 1/3 cup plus 2 tablespoons olive oil
- 1 cup finely chopped fennel
- 1 cup finely chopped leeks (white and light green parts only)
- 4 large garlic cloves, minced
- 1/2 cup dry white wine
- 1 tablespoon tomato paste
- 1 pound tomatoes, peeled, seeded, chopped
- 1/2 cup chopped drained oil-packed sun-dried tomatoes
- 1/3 cup pitted sliced kalamata olives or other brine-cured black olives
- 4 teaspoons minced fresh rosemary
- 4 6-ounce halibut fillets (each about 1 inch thick)

- lemon wedges and leftover fennel fronds for garnish

Direction

- Heat 2 tablespoons oil in heavy large skillet over medium-high heat. Add fennel, leeks, and garlic and sauté until crisp-tender, about 5 minutes. Add wine and cook until reduced by half, about 3 minutes. Add tomato paste, both kinds of tomatoes, the olives and 1 teaspoon of the rosemary and cook until slightly thickened. Season to taste with salt and pepper. (This part can be made ahead - up to 2 days. Rewarm over low heat before serving.
- Combine remaining 1/3 cup oil and 3 teaspoons rosemary in small bowl. In a shallow dish arrange halibut in a single layer. Pour flavored oil over; cover and refrigerate at least 1 hour and up to 4 hours.
- Prepare grill to medium-high heat. Season halibut with salt and pepper. Grill until fish is just opaque in center, about 7 minutes total, turning once.
- Arrange fish on serving platter; spoon relish over.
- Garnish with lemon wedges and the fennel fronds.

155. Halibut With Lemon Shallots And Herbs Recipe

Serving: 4 | Prep: | Cook: 15mins | Ready in:

Ingredients

- ¼ cup butter
- 2 tsp finely chopped shallots, or fresh chives
- 2 tsp finely chopped tarragon or dill
- 2 tsp finely chopped fresh parsley
- ½ tsp Dijon mustard
- ½ tsp lemon
- ¼ tsp crushed garlic
- 4 fillets (6 0z) halibut or sea bass

Direction

- In small bowl, mix together the butter, shallots, tarragon, parsley, mustard, lemon juice and garlic until well combined.
- Broil the fish for 4 - 6 minutes per side, or until it flakes from the center with a fork.
- Spread about 1 tbsp. of the spread mixture over each portion of fish.
- Garnish with a couple of sprigs of chives.

156. Halibut With Red Pepper And Olive Relish Recipe

Serving: 4 | Prep: | Cook: 20mins | Ready in:

Ingredients

- 3 tablespoons olive oil
- 1 1/2 cups coarsely chopped redbell pepper
- 1/2 cup chopped red onion
- 3 large garlic cloves, chopped
- 1 tablespoon chopped fresh thyme
- 1/2 cup coarsely chopped pimiento-stuffed green olives
- 1 tablespoon balsamic vinegar
- 1 tablespoon tomato paste
- cayenne pepper
- 4 8- to 10-ounce halibut fillets
- fresh thyme sprigs

Direction

- Preheat oven to 375°F. Brush large rimmed baking sheet with olive oil. Heat 3 tablespoons oil in large skillet over medium-high heat. Add bell pepper, onion, garlic, and thyme. Sauté until bell pepper is soft, about 6 minutes. Remove from heat. Mix in olives, vinegar, and tomato paste. Season relish to taste with cayenne, salt, and pepper.
- Place fish on prepared baking sheet and brush with olive oil. Sprinkle with salt and pepper. Spoon enough relish over each fillet to cover. Reserve remaining relish. Bake fish until just

opaque in center, about 10 minutes. Transfer fish to serving platter. Garnish with thyme sprigs; serve with reserved relish.

157. Halibut With Sour Cream Dill Sauce Recipe

Serving: 4 | Prep: | Cook: 15mins | Ready in:

Ingredients

- 4 - 6 oz halibut fillets
- 2 tbsp. olive oil
- course salt
- 2/3 c. sour cream
- 2 tbsp. red onion, finely chopped
- 1/2 tsp. finely shredded lemon peel
- 1 tsp. fresh dillweed or 1/2 tsp. dried dillweed

Direction

- Preheat oven to 450 degrees.
- Rinse fish under cool running water to wash away impurities. Pat dry with paper towels and rub with a bit of olive oil or melted butter. Sprinkle with coarse salt and pepper. Set aside.
- Prepare sour cream-dill sauce by combining sour cream, red onion (or chives), lemon peel and dill weed. (Use a good, full fat sour cream for this). Set sauce aside.
- Place halibut fillets in shallow pan and roast in oven for 6 to 8 minutes, depending on thickness, or until fish flakes easily with fork.
- Spoon the sour cream mixture over each fillet. Bake 8 -10 minutes longer, or until the sour cream is set. Garnish with thin lemon slices and parsley.

158. Halibut With A Creamy Dijon Sauce Recipe

Serving: 4 | Prep: | Cook: 15mins | Ready in:

Ingredients

- 4 halibut - about 1 in. thick
- olive oil for brushing
- salt and pepper
- few sprigs fresh parsley
- lemon slices to serve
- mustard Sauce
- 4 Tbsp. Dijon mustard
- 1 cup heavy cream
- 1/2 tsp. sugar
- 1 Tbsp. fresh lemon juice
- 1 teas. dried tarragon

Direction

- Heat the grill to medium. Spray Pam or oil the grill grates. Season the halibut with salt and pepper and brush with oil. Make sure grill grates are hot before putting halibut on or it will stick. Grill for about 5-7 minutes per side - season and brush with oil when you turn them.
- Meanwhile, make your Dijon sauce by putting all the ingredients into a saucepan. Stir constantly while the mixture comes almost to a boil. It will thicken slightly and then remove it from the heat. Taste and adjust seasoning if you wish.
- Serve the fish steaks with the sauce over and lemon wedges.

159. Hawaiian Halibut Recipe

Serving: 2 | Prep: | Cook: 40mins | Ready in:

Ingredients

- 2 cups cooked rice
- 4 teaspoons lemon juice

- 1/2 cup melted butter
- 1 teaspoon seasoned salt
- 1/2 teaspoon curry powder
- 1 can pineapple chunks drained
- 2 halibut steaks
- 1 lemon for garnish

Direction

- Combine rice, 3 teaspoons lemon juice, 1/4 cup butter, curry powder and about 2/3 pineapple chunks.
- Sprinkle each steak with 1/2 teaspoon lemon juice and 1/2 teaspoon seasoning salt.
- Place 1 steak in a large shallow pan and brush with 1 tablespoon butter and press rice filling on top.
- Top with other steak then brush with butter and secure with skewers.
- Spoon extra rice around steaks and bake at 350 for 40 minutes.
- Garnish with pineapple chunks and lemon wedges.

160. Healthy Fish Tacos 2 Avocado Creama Recipe

Serving: 4 | Prep: | Cook: 20mins | Ready in:

Ingredients

- 1lb Tilapia or other firm white fish
- 2tbls all purpose flour
- olive oil
- white wine(optional)
- 1 tbls chili powder
- 1tbls cumin
- 1tsp oregano
- 1tsp salt
- 1tsp pepper
- 2 cloves garlic, pressed or chopped
- 8 corn tortillas
- 2 cups coleslaw mix
- 1 bunch green onions, chopped
- 1 lime
- 1 avocado
- 1/2 cup light sour cream
- 1/4 cup light mayo
- 1tsp red wine vinegar
- 1 tbls cilantro, chopped
- salt and pepper to taste

Direction

- Mix flour, chili powder, cumin, oregano, salt and pepper.
- Rub mixture on both sides of fish fillet.
- Pour a tbsp of olive oil in a non-stick skillet, heat.
- Cook fish on both sides till light and flakey.
- Deglaze pan with white wine (optional).
- Chop green onions, mix with coleslaw mix.
- Make creama.
- Mash avocado, cilantro, juice of one lime, sour cream and mayo.
- Add vinegar, add salt and pepper to taste.
- Heat corn tortillas over gas flame or in skillet. Take 2 corn tortillas, add some fish, coleslaw mix and top with creama. Enjoy.
- For a low carb option, can also be served over a salad.

161. Heavenly Baked Haddock Recipe

Serving: 4 | Prep: | Cook: 20mins | Ready in:

Ingredients

- 1 1/2 lbs fresh or thawed haddock, cut into 2 fillets
- 1 cup New England style oyster crackers
- 1/2 stick butter melted
- ocean fish seasoning or salt and pepper
- fresh lemon
- mayonnaise , about T tbs
- gongonzolla blue cheese
- paprika

Direction

- Preheat oven to 425F.
- Coarse crumble crackers and then pour the butter over and mix till very well combined.
- Squeeze juice from a fresh lemon over fish and then season fish.
- Using enough mayo, spread evenly over fish.
- Press cracker mixture over fillets.
- Lay some slices of gorgonzola across the top of each fillet.
- Sprinkle with paprika.
- Bake fish until topping is golden and fish is cooked and done.
- Carefully split the 2 portions into 4 pieces.
- I find this easier to prepare instead of 4 smaller pieces.
- Serve at once.

162. Heavenly Halibut Recipe

Serving: 3 | Prep: | Cook: 10mins | Ready in:

Ingredients

- 3T grated parmesan cheese
- 3T butter, softened
- 1 1/2t Mayo
- 2 1/2t lemon juice
- 1 1/4T green onions
- 1/8t salt
- 1t (or more) hot pepper sauce
- 3/4-1lb skinless halibut fillets

Direction

- Preheat Broiler. Grease baking dish.
- Mix Parmesan, butter, mayo, lemon juice, onions, salt, & hot pepper sauce.
- Arrange Halibut in prepared baking dish.
- Broil Halibut filets 8 minutes or until easily flaked with a fork.
- Spread with Parmesan mixture and continue broiling for 2 minutes or until topping is bubbly and lightly browned.

163. Herb Crusted Halibut With Potatoes And Artichokes Recipe

Serving: 4 | Prep: | Cook: 35mins | Ready in:

Ingredients

- vegetable Spray
- 3 large red potatoes (about 1 pound), unpeeled, cut into 1/8-inch slices
- 1/4 tsp. pepper
- 1/4 C fat-free or light mayonnaise
- 2 Tbl. chopped fresh rosemary or 2 tsp. dried, crushed
- 2 Tbl. chopped fresh thyme, or 2 tsp. dried, crumbled
- 1 Tbl. chopped fresh oregano, or 1 tsp. dried, crumbled
- 4 halibut or salmon fillets (about 4 ounces each)
- 14.5-ounce can artichoke quarters, rinsed and drained
- 1 C halved Cherry Toamtoes
- 1 Tbl. fresh lemon juice
- 2 tsp. olive oil

Direction

- Preheat oven to 400 degrees.
- Lightly spray a rimmed baking sheet with vegetable oil spray.
- Arrange the potatoes in a single layer. Lightly spray with vegetable oil spray. Sprinkle with the pepper.
- Bake for 18 to 20 minutes (no stirring needed), or until the potatoes are tender and lightly browned.
- Meanwhile, in a small bowl, stir together the mayonnaise, rosemary, thyme, and oregano. Cover and refrigerate while the potatoes bake or for up to 8 hours.
- Rinse the fish and pat dry with paper towels.

- Arrange the fish about 2 inches apart on the cooked potatoes.
- Scatter the artichokes and tomatoes over the potatoes.
- Drizzle the lemon juice and oil over the vegetables.
- Lightly spray over the tops of the vegetables with vegetable oil spray.
- Spoon the mayonnaise mixture over the tops and sides of the fillets.
- Bake for 12 to 15 minutes, or until the fish flakes easily when tested with a fork and the vegetables are warmed through.

164. Hoisin Baked Salmon Recipe

Serving: 2 | Prep: | Cook: 10mins | Ready in:

Ingredients

- 2 (6 ounce) salmon, pieces
- 2 tablespoons hoisin sauce
- 2 teaspoons soy sauce
- 5 drops dark sesame oil
- 1/4 teaspoon chili paste (optional) or hot sauce (optional)
- 1-2 teaspoon sesame seeds (light or black)

Direction

- Preheat oven to 375 degrees.
- Place salmon on baking dish or tray.
- Thin hoisin with a little soy sauce and flavor with a few drops of sesame oil.
- Stir in chili paste, if desired.
- Brush or spoon mixture on salmon.
- Sprinkle with sesame seeds.
- Bake for 8 to 10 minutes, or until it flakes with a fork.
- Makes 2 servings.
- Serve with rice or pasta that has been tossed with a little sesame oil, and steamed green vegetables like broccoli, bok choy or green beans, drizzled with bottled oyster sauce.

165. Honey Ginger Grilled Salmon Recipe

Serving: 4 | Prep: | Cook: 15mins | Ready in:

Ingredients

- 1 teaspoon ground ginger
- 1 teaspoon garlic powder
- 1/2 cup soy sauce
- 1/3 cup orange juice
- 1/4 cup honey
- 1 green onion, chopped
- 1 1/2 pounds salmon fillets (4 6 oz. fillets)

Direction

- In a large zip top plastic bag, combine first 6 ingredients; mix well.
- Place salmon in bag and seal tightly.
- Turn bag gently to distribute marinade.
- Refrigerate 15 minutes or up to 30 minutes for stronger flavor.
- Turn bag occasionally.
- Lightly grease cold grill rack.
- Preheat grill for medium heat.
- Remove salmon from marinade; reserved marinade.
- Grill 12 to 15 minutes per inch of thickness or until fish flakes easily with fork.
- Brush with reserved marinade up until the last 5 minutes of cooking time.
- Discard leftover marinade.
- Serves 4

166. Honey Ginger Salmon Recipe

Serving: 4 | Prep: | Cook: 15mins | Ready in:

Ingredients

- 1/3c orange juice
- 1/3c soy sauce
- 1/4c honey
- 1tsp. ground ginger
- 1tsp garlic powder
- 1 green onion
- 4 6oz. salmon fillets

Direction

- In a small bowl, combine orange juice, soy sauce, honey, ground ginger, garlic powder and green onion. Place salmon in a large glass dish and pour marinade over them. Turn to coat and refrigerate 15 mins.
- Preheat grill. Discard marinade and grill salmon over med-high heat for 6-8 mins a side or till fish flakes easily with a fork.

167. Horseradish Asiago Encrusted Salmon Recipe

Serving: 6 | Prep: | Cook: 15mins | Ready in:

Ingredients

- 4-6 oz. skinless salmon fillets
- 3/4 C fresh shredded horseradish root
- 3/4 C shredded asiago cheese
- 1/4 C butter (melted)
- 1/4 C olive oil
- salt
- pepper
- 2 tsp. minced fresh rosemary
- 1 lemon
- Grated parmesan for garnish
- Sauce
- 1 C sour cream
- 1 bunch cilantro
- 1/4 tsp. ground coriander

Direction

- Mince 2 tbsp. fresh cilantro, reserve remaining cilantro for garnish. Combine sour cream, cilantro, and coriander.
- Mix well and set aside.
- In a bowl combine grated horseradish, asiago, butter and rosemary.
- Brush each salmon fillet with olive oil then a dash of salt and pepper.
- Coat with asiago cheese mixture
- Place each fillet on a well-oiled baking sheet and bake at 350 until golden brown (about 15 minutes)
- Remove and garnish with sour cream mixture, fresh squeezed lemon and cilantro leaves.
- Dust with parmesan and enjoy!

168. Horseradish Crusted Cod With Lemon Roasted Potatoes Recipe

Serving: 4 | Prep: | Cook: 60mins | Ready in:

Ingredients

- 1 1/4 lb red-skinned baby potatoes, scrubbed and sliced very thinly, about 1/8 inch (about 4 potatoes)
- 1 lemon wedge, about 1/4 lemon. thinly sliced widthwise, discarding seeds and ends
- 1 Tbl olive oil
- 3 garlic cloves. minced and divided
- 1 tsp kosher salt, divided
- 1/2 tsp freshly ground black pepper, divided
- 3/4 C panko crumbs
- 2 Tbl minced fresh parsley, divided
- 3 Tbl drained prepared horseradish, divided
- 3Tbl reduced fat mayonnaise
- 1 Tbl Dijon mustard
- 1 Tbl lemon juice
- 4 Skinless cod fillets, about 6ounces each, 1 1/4 to 1 1/2 inches thick

Direction

- Adjust oven rack to upper third position and preheat oven to 425F
- Spray a 9 x13 baking dish with cooking spray
- Add potatoes, lemon slices, olive oil, 2 cloves of the garlic, 1/2 tsp. salt and 1/4 tsp. black pepper and spread around the baking dish so potatoes are evenly layered
- Roast at 425F for 40 minutes, turning potatoes with a spatula after 20 minutes
- While potatoes are cooking, toss breadcrumbs with 1 tbsp. of the parsley and 1tbsp. of the horseradish in a small bowl
- In a separate bowl, mix remaining ingredients, except for salt and pepper
- Pat cod dry with paper towels and then season with remaining 1/2 tsp. salt and 1/4 tsp. pepper
- Brush tops and sides with mayonnaise mixture and sprinkle and press breadcrumbs into mayonnaise
- After the potatoes have cooked for 40 minutes, place fillets on top of potatoes, return to oven and cook another 13 to 17 minutes or until fish flakes easily when prodded with a paring knife
- Serve immediately from the baking dish
- Note: if ends of fillets are small, fold under to make fish as uniform as possible in thickness

169. Horseradish Salmon Recipe

Serving: 4 | Prep: | Cook: 8mins | Ready in:

Ingredients

- 1 english cucumber,cut in half lengthwise and then in 1/4" thick half-moons
- 2 Tbs. white vinegar
- 2 Tbs chopped fresh dill
- 2 Tbs olive oil
- 1/2 c panko
- 2 Tbs prepared horseradish,drained
- 4 skinless,boneless salmon fillets(5 to 6 oz ea.)
- 6 oz. baby spinach

Direction

- In large bowl, toss cucumber, vinegar, 1 Tbsp. dill, 1 Tbsp. oil and 1/8 tsp each salt and pepper.
- In small bowl, combine panko, horseradish and remaining dill and oil. Sprinkle salmon with 1/8 tsp. each salt and pepper; place on cookie sheet, smooth side up. Press panko mixture evenly on top of fillets. Bake salmon 8 mins or till golden brown on top and opaque throughout.
- Toss spinach with cucumber mixture in bowl, serve with salmon.

170. Hot Grilled Trout Recipe

Serving: 8 | Prep: | Cook: 10mins | Ready in:

Ingredients

- 1/4 cup lemon juice
- 2 tablespoons margarine melted
- 2 tablespoons vegetable oil
- 2 tablespoons parsley chopped
- 2 tablespoons sesame seeds
- 1 tablespoon Tabasco
- 1/2 teaspoon ground ginger
- 1/2 teaspoon salt
- 4 trout about 1 pound each

Direction

- In shallow dish combine juice, margarine, oil, parsley, seeds, Tabasco, ginger and salt.
- Mix well then pierce skin of fish in several places with tines of fork.
- Roll fish in juice mixture to coat inside and out then cover and refrigerate 1 hour.
- Turn occasionally then remove fish from marinade and reserve marinade.
- Place fish in handheld hinged grill then brush fish with reserved marinade.

- Cook 4" from hot coals for 5 minutes.
- Turn and brush with marinade then cook 5 minutes longer.

171. Hot N Spicy Catfish Strips Recipe

Serving: 6 | Prep: | Cook: 15mins | Ready in:

Ingredients

- 2 pounds of catfish fillets strips
- 2 jalapeno chili, finely minced
- 1 c. cornmeal
- 1/4 tsp salt
- 2 garlic cloves, finely minced
- canola oil
- salsa and lime wedges

Direction

- Rinse catfish and pat dry (strips should be just moist enough for coating to stick. Combine cornmeal, jalapenos, garlic and salt in a large zip lock bag. Add catfish strips and shake until all are coated.
- Heat about 1 to 1-½ inches of oil in a large skillet over medium high heat. Place coated catfish in hot oil, turn when brown. Continue to fry until both sides are brown and the fish begins to flake when pierced with a fork.
- Remove and drain on paper towels to remove excess oil.
- Serve with salsa and lime wedges.

172. How To Cook Bouillabaisse In Marseilles Or Anywhere Else Recipe

Serving: 8 | Prep: | Cook: 2mins | Ready in:

Ingredients

- • 3.5 kg firm, white fleshed fish; Pick 3 or 4 from Snapper, Rockfish, Monkfish, cod, Grouper, halibut, haddock, Ocean Catfish, Blackfish, etc.
- • 2 kg "oily" fish; Pick 2 from Bluefish, Moray eel, Conger eel, mackerel, dogfish, striped bass, sea bass, Spanish mackerel, mahimahi (dolphinfish).
- • 2.5 - 3kg Whole Main lobster; large shrimp may be used for part of this.
- • 1 - 1.5kg mussels in their shell.
- • 2kg small clams, in their shell.
- • 5 Tbs butter
- • 2 med. yellow onions peeled & sliced
- • 8 - 10 cups water
- • 2 bouquet garni each with 4 sprigs fresh parsley, 6 sprigs fresh thyme, 10 black peppercorns, and 1 bay leaf, tied in cheesecloth
- • 1 cup dry white wine (decent stuff please)
- • 1 ½ cups olive oil (extra virgin is okay but regular has more flavor)
- • 6 - 8 large garlic cloves, finely chopped (to taste)
- • A pinch of saffron stepped in ¼ cup hot water until needed
- • ½ tsp saffron threads stepped in tepid dry white wine until needed
- • 1 large yellow onion, finely chopped.
- • 3 leeks, white and light green part only, halved lengthwise, and thinly sliced.
- • 3 stalks celery, finely chopped.
- • 2 pounds ripe plum tomatoes, peeled, seeded and chopped
- • 1 long thin strip of orange zest, no pith
- • 1 Tbs fennel seed
- • salt and freshly ground pepper to taste.
- • boiling water as needed
- • 2 Tbs tomato past
- • 2 Tbs anis flavored liquor, Pernod or ouzo
- • ½ cup fresh parsley leaves, finely chopped.
- • 1 Sauce rouille (see Sauce Rouille)

Direction

- 1. Gut, scale and clean the fish. Save the heads, tails and carcasses. If the fish monger has them, get them back. Cut the fish into 2 X 4" pieces and set aside.

- 2. Prepare the fish broth. Rinse the fish heads, tails, and carcasses in cold water. Break the carcasses into pieces. In a large stockpot, melt the butter, then cook the sliced onions until soft but not brown, stirring occasionally. Add the fish heads and bones and cover with the cold water. Put in one of the bouquet garni and the wine. Bring to a boil, then reduce the heat to low, cover with lid tilted and simmer for 2 hours, skimming occasionally. Strain the fish broth through a conical strainer and set aside to cool. Discard all the fish bits. You should have 10 cups of fish broth when finished. Clean the stockpot for later use.
- 3. As soon as you get the fish broth going, marinate the fish in a large ceramic or glass bowl with 1/4 cup of the olive oil, half of the chopped garlic, and the saffron threads for 2 hours in the refrigerator.
- 4. Place the mussels and clams in very cold fresh water to soak and purge a bit. Beard the muscles.
- 5. Boil the Lobster, and if using shrimp as usual and set aside to cool. When cool remove lobster tails from shell, devein and cut into 2" X 2" pieces. Shell and devein the shrimp. If you don't know how to do this you're on the wrong page.
- 6. In the large stockpot, heat the remaining 1 1/4 cups olive oil over medium heat, then cook the chopped onions, leeks, and celery for 15 minutes, stirring often. Add the tomatoes, the remaining garlic, the remaining bouquet garni, the orange zest, and fennel seeds. Stir in the reserved fish broth and the saffron steeped in wine and season with a little salt and pepper Remember that the clams and mussels will add salt to the dish when they are added. Bring to a boil, then reduce the heat to medium-low and simmer for 40 minutes. The broth can be left over very low heat, covered, for hours. If you're going to rest a while put the lobster and shrimp in the fridge.
- 7. When you are ready to prepare the final stages of the bouillabaisse, bring the broth back to a furious, rolling boil. Keep the broth boiling furiously so the oil emulsifies. Add the oily fish and boil, uncovered, over very high heat for 8 minutes. Shake the pot to prevent sticking. Now put the firm-fleshed white fish, lobster, muscles & clams in and boil hard for 6 minutes. Add more boiling water if necessary to cover the fish. Shake the casserole or pot occasionally. Mix the tomato paste and anise liqueur.
- 8. Carefully remove the fish, lobster, shrimp, calms and muscles from the broth with a slotted spoon and spatula or skimmer and transfer to a large bowl or deep platter.
- 9. Strain the broth through a fine mesh strainer into a soup tureen or large bowl, discarding what doesn't go through. Whisk in the tomato paste-and-anise mixture. Add the fish, lobster, clams and mussels to the broth and serve with the croutes and sauce rouille on separate plates.
- By Jove, I think you've got it. Bon for sure Apatite.

173. Indian Broiled Fish With Spices Recipe

Serving: 4 | Prep: | Cook: 15mins | Ready in:

Ingredients

- 2 tablespoons lemon juice
- 2 tablespoons dry mustard
- 2 teaspoons ground cumin
- 1 teaspoon ground coriander
- 1 teaspoon salt
- 1/4 teaspoon garam masala
- 4 halibut steaks
- 2 tablespoons melted butter

Direction

- Mix together all ingredients except fish and butter.

- Spread mixture evenly on both sides of fish then place fish in shallow glass dish.
- Cover and refrigerate at least 12 hours.
- Set oven control to broil and arrange fish on rack in broiler pan and drizzle with butter.
- Broil with tops 4" from heat until light brown about 7 minutes then turn.
- Drizzle with melted butter then broil 7 minutes longer.

174. Indian Fried Fish Gujurati Style Recipe

Serving: 6 | Prep: | Cook: 10mins | Ready in:

Ingredients

- 1and 1/2 pounds boneless fish fillets of your choice (we like tilapia)
- 2 Tablesps. besan (chick-pea flour. Found in Indo/Pak grocery stores)
- 2 Tablesps. white flour
- 1/2 teacup warm water
- 1 and 1/2 cups vegetable oil (for frying)
- 1 and 1/2 teasp. salt
- 1 teaspoon garam masala
- 2 Tablesps. fresh cilantro; chopped
- 1 Tablespoon white vinegar
- 1/2 teaspoon cayenne powder (or to taste)

Direction

- 1) Wash & cut fillets in half. Place on large plate & sprinkle them with 1 teaspoon salt, 1/2 teaspoon garam masala & the vinegar. Let sit while you make the batter.
- 2) For batter: Combine chick-pea flour & white flour together in a fairly large bowl. Make into a thick batter by adding the water gradually & beating well. Add the remaining salt & garam masala, herbs & cayenne powder to batter & beat for several minutes. Heat oil in deep frying pan until it's quite hot. Coat fillet pieces on both sides with the batter. Slide 3 or 4 pieces at a time, carefully, into hot oil (don't crowd pan) & fry fairly quickly (so fillets don't absorb too much oil) until golden. Remove with slotted spoon, letting excess oil drain back into pan. Place on paper towels for minute or two before arranging on serving platter. This dish is traditionally served with lemon pickle & curried potatoes & tomatoes.

175. Indian Spiced Roast Salmon Recipe

Serving: 4 | Prep: | Cook: 15mins | Ready in:

Ingredients

- 1 teaspoon ground cumin
- 1 teaspoon ground coriander
- 1/2 teaspoon ground turmeric
- 1/2 teaspoon dried thyme
- 1/2 teaspoon fennel seeds, crushed
- 1/2 teaspoon black pepper
- 1/4 teaspoon ground cinnamon
- 1/8 teaspoon ground cloves
- 4 (6-ounce) salmon fillets (about 1 1.4-inches thick)
- 1/2 teaspoon olive oil
- 1/4 cup plain fat-free yogurt
- 4 lemon wedges

Direction

- Heat oven to 400.
- Combine first 8 ingredients in a shallow dish. Sprinkle fillets with salt, dredge fillets in spice mixture. Heat oil in a large skillet over medium-high heat. Add fillets, skin side up; cook 5 minutes or until bottoms are golden. Turn fillets over. Wrap handle of skillet with foil; bake at 400 for 10 minutes or until fish flakes easily when tested with a fork. Remove skin from fillets; discard skin. Serve with yogurt and lemon wedges.

176. Italian Sole For Your Soul Recipe

Serving: 6 | Prep: | Cook: 20mins | Ready in:

Ingredients

- 2 1/2 lbs fillet of sole
- 1/4 c olive oil
- 1 clove garlic flattened
- 1/4 c diced onion
- 3 tbl diced green pepper
- 1/4 c diced celery
- 1 1/2 c crushed tomatoes
- 1/4 c sherry wine
- 1 bay leaf
- 2 tbl diced prosciutto
- 3 tbl grated parmesan cheese
- 1 c bread crumbs
- 3 tbl butter
- salt and freshly ground pepper

Direction

- Heat the oil and brown the garlic-discard garlic.
- Sauté diced onions, peppers and celery for 5 minutes.
- Add tomatoes, wine, bay leaf, salt and pepper.
- Place sauce in a casserole dish with the fish on top.
- Mix the prosciutto, cheese, and breadcrumbs together and sprinkle on top of the filets.
- Break up the butter and put on top of the fish.
- Bake for 20 minutes at 375 degrees.

177. Japanese Grilled Tuna Recipe

Serving: 4 | Prep: | Cook: 5mins | Ready in:

Ingredients

- 1 tbsp sesame oil
- 1 tbsp vegetable oil
- 1 tbsp grated ginger
- 1 tbsp cracked black pepper
- 4 eight-ounce tuna steaks about 1 inch thick
- ---------------------------
- wasabi soy sauce Glaze:
- 1/2 cup granulated sugar
- 1/2 cup water
- 1/2 cup rice vinegar
- 1/4 cup light soy sauce
- 4 slices fresh ginger, smashed
- 2 tsp wasabi powder
- salt

Direction

- Combine oils, ginger, and pepper; brush on the tuna steaks.
- Sprinkle with salt.
- Marinate for 30 minutes.
- Combine sugar, water, rice vinegar, soy sauce, and vinegar.
- Bring to a boil on high heat, and reduce until syrupy (about 15 minutes).
- Whisk in Wasabi paste.
- The glaze should be used at room temperature.
- Grill tuna 2 minutes per side, with the lid closed for 'very rare' or, grill 3 to 4 minutes per side for 'medium-rare'.
- Drizzle glaze over the fish.

178. Jetts Salmon Patties Recipe

Serving: 5 | Prep: | Cook: 20mins | Ready in:

Ingredients

- 1- 2 cans good quality salmon (15 oz)
- 1/2 small onion chopped(optional)
- 1 egg
- worcestershire sauce
- Franks hot sauce
- Ritz crackers(1/2 sleeve or more)

- baggie for crushing crackers
- seasoned salt
- pepper
- garlic powder
- oil for frying

Direction

- Drain juice out of the salmon can.
- Pour salmon into a bowl and remove the skin and the bones.
- With a fork, break up the salmon.
- Add seasonings to your liking. You can taste it before adding the egg to make sure it's not too salty.
- Add crackers to the baggie and crush up.
- After you have seasoned the salmon to your liking, add the egg and cracker crumbs. The consistency should not be too sticky. You should be able to spoon out the mixture and make patties.
- Have your oil hot in a large cast iron skillet.
- Carefully, carefully add the salmon patties into the hot oil and let brown on one side before turning over. Have a plate with paper towels ready to put patties on after they are removed from oil.
- *** Swallowing your pride seldom leads to indigestion ***

179. Jewel Studded Salmon With Cilantro Cream Cheese Recipe

Serving: 4 | Prep: | Cook: 10mins | Ready in:

Ingredients

- 2 large salmon filets, skinned
- 2 cloves garlic
- 4 tablespoons softened cream cheese
- 4 stalks of fresh cilantro, chopped
- 1-teaspoon kosher salt

Direction

- Peel and mince the garlic.
- Mince the cilantro.
- Thoroughly mix the garlic, cilantro, and cream cheese, and then set aside.
- Butterfly the salmon filets.
- Spread the cream cheese mixture into the salmon and fold it back up.
- Place on hot grill and cook for about 6 minutes on each side.
- Sprinkle with salt during cooking.

180. Kitchen Disaster Salmon With Lemon Herb Sauce Recipe

Serving: 4 | Prep: | Cook: 20mins | Ready in:

Ingredients

- 3 shallots, very finely chopped
- 1 1/2 oz. butter
- Zest and juice of 1 1/2 lemons
- 1 1/2 generous teaspoons garlic powder
- 1 1/2 generous teaspoons onion powder
- 2 1/2 generous teaspoons Italian style dried herb mix
- 1 1/2 pints hot chicken stock
- 1 1/2 generous teaspoons chicken bouillon granules
- juice of another lemon, a smallish one
- 1 1/2 generous teaspoon cornstarch
- 1 1/2 tablespoons parsley, finely chopped
- More chicken stock if needed
- 2 tablespoons bland flavoured oil (I used groundnut)
- 4 good sized salmon fillets
- lemon wedges to serve
- parsley to garnish

Direction

- Heat butter in a frying pan.
- Add the shallots and sauté gently until soft but not browned, about 5-7 minutes.

- Add lemon zest and stir in well. Cook briefly.
- Add the garlic powder, onion powder and dried herbs. Stir in well and cook gently for half a minute or so.
- Add the lemon juice and chicken stock, and add the bouillon granules. Stir well, turn up the heat and reduce the liquid a bit.
- Transfer to a saucepan. Bring back up to the simmer.
- Make a slurry with the lemon juice and the cornstarch. Add to the sauce and cook until thickened.
- Add the parsley and stir well in.
- Turn off the heat and set aside while cooking the salmon.
- Wipe out the frying pan.
- Add the oil and heat.
- Put in the salmon fillets and pan fry on a low-medium heat, turning once, till just done - about 15-20 minutes total depending on thickness.
- Cook your veg of choice.
- Just before salmon is ready to serve, reheat the sauce. Add more stock if it is too thick.
- Put the salmon on the plates and pour over the fish juices from the pan. Then pour over the sauce.
- Serve with plain boiled new potatoes and veg of choice, and garnish with lemon wedge and parsley.
- Then get someone else to do the washing-up.

181. LOUP DE MERR AU FENOUIL STRIPED BASS WITH FENNEL Recipe

Serving: 8 | Prep: | Cook: 20mins | Ready in:

Ingredients

- 2 two pound striped bass
- flour
- vegetable oil
- Dried fennel branches
- 4 garlic cloves minced
- 1 tablespoon minced parsley
- toasted bread crumbs
- Coarsely minced hardboiled eggs
- Sauce:
- 1 glass of dry white wine
- 1/2 teaspoon salt
- 1 teaspoon freshly ground black pepper
- 1 teaspoon fennel seed
- 1 cup fish stock

Direction

- Clean and split fish.
- Coat lightly in flour and sauté in hot oil until golden brown on both sides.
- Place in 350 oven for 15 minutes.
- Remove fish from oven and arrange on bed of fennel branches in an oven dish.
- Cover with minced garlic, parsley, bread crumbs and hard boiled eggs.
- To make sauce combine all ingredients and simmer 15 minutes.
- Pour sauce over fish and return to oven for 10 minutes.

182. Lemon And Wine Fish Recipe

Serving: 6 | Prep: | Cook: 30mins | Ready in:

Ingredients

- 2 lemons,divided
- 6 halibut steaks or tilapia fillers (about 1-1/2 lbs)
- 2 Tbs olive oil
- 2 Tbs white wine
- 2 cloves garlic,peeled and minced
- 1/4 c chopped scallions
- 2 Tbs chopped fresh parsley

Direction

- Heat grill. Cut six 10" squares of heavy-duty aluminum foil. Zest juice of 1 lemon; trim and slice remaining lemon. In med. bowl, whisk together olive oil, 3 tbsp lemon juice, 2 tsp lemon zest, white wine and garlic until blended. Stir in chopped scallions and parsley.
- Season tilapia or halibut with salt and ground black pepper, if desired. Place 1 piece of fish in center of each foil square.
- Pour lemon-oil mixture evenly over fish. Top with lemon slices. Fold foil over fish and press to seal edges tightly. Grill 8 mins or till fish flakes with fork. Garnish with fresh parsley, if desired.

183. Lemon Crusted Baked Halibut Recipe

Serving: 4 | Prep: | Cook: 25mins | Ready in:

Ingredients

- 4 halibut fillets (4-8 oz. each)
- 1/4 c. lemon juice or 4-8 packets TrueLemon*
- 4 tsp. olive oil
- 2 tbsp. plain dried breadcrumbs
- lemon pepper seasoning
- salt
- fresh ground pepper
- 1/4 c. parsley

Direction

- Preheat oven to 350
- Spray baking pan with non-stick olive oil cooking spray
- Rinse fillets in cool water, paper towel lightly to dry
- Place fillets skin-side down on pan
- Drizzle lemon juice onto fillets or sprinkle them with TrueLemon*
- Brush with the olive oil and dust a little lemon pepper seasoning on the fillets
- Pat breadcrumbs, salt and pepper and a little more lemon pepper seasoning onto fillets, making a light crust with the breadcrumbs and seasoning
- Bake fish for 20-30 minutes until it's nice and flaky
- Add leftover lemon juice to the fish, spooning any juice in pan back onto fish
- Season with more salt & pepper and lemon pepper seasoning if you desire (I sometimes like extra lemon pepper seasoning on mine!)
- Garnish with parsley
- Enjoy!
- NOTE: *TrueLemon is a crystallized lemon juice. I use it along with fresh lemon juice sometimes. But it certainly suffices alone. Because of how quickly produce goes bad & the fact that I tend to make this dish on a whim, it's a great option for me! For the purists out there, I just wanted to say it's 100% pure, natural lemon juice/oils that have been crystallized. Nothing else. I love it because it is all natural, contains no artificial flavors or sweeteners, no preservatives or sodium, has 0 calories, contains Vitamin C, & is easy to use, especially when you're out of fresh lemons! One packet = 1 wedge of lemon.

184. Lemon Garlic Tilapia Recipe

Serving: 4 | Prep: | Cook: 40mins | Ready in:

Ingredients

- 4 tilapia fillets
- 3 Tbsp. fresh lemon juice
- 1 Tbsp. butter, melted
- 1 clove of garlic, finely chopped
- 1 tsp. dried parsley flakes
- pepper to taste

Direction

- Preheat the oven to 375 degrees.
- Spray baking dish with cooking spray.

- Rinse tilapia fillets under cool water, and pat dry with paper towels.
- Place fillets in baking dish.
- Pour lemon juice over the fillets
- Drizzle with butter on top.
- Sprinkle with garlic, parsley and pepper.
- Bake for about 30 minutes until flaky when pulled apart with a fork.

185. Lemon Glazed Salmon Fillet Recipe

Serving: 6 | Prep: | Cook: 30mins | Ready in:

Ingredients

- 1 1/2 c. brown sugar
- 6 Tbsp. butter or marg., melted
- 3 to 6 Tbsp. lemon juice
- 2 1/4 tsp. dill weed
- 3/4 tsp. cayenne pepper
- ______________
- 1 salmon fillet (about 2 pounds)
- lemon-pepper seasoning

Direction

- Small bowl- Combine first 5 ingredients; mix well.
- Remove 1/2 c. to saucepan; simmer until heated through.
- Set aside remaining for basting.
- ______________
- Sprinkle salmon with lemon pepper.
- Place on grill with skin side down.
- Grill covered, medium heat, 5 mins.
- Brush with reserved brown sugar mixture.
- Grill 10-15 mins. longer, basting occasionally.
- ______________
- Serve with warm sauce.

186. Lemon Grilled Tilapia Recipe

Serving: 4 | Prep: | Cook: 15mins | Ready in:

Ingredients

- 8-10 bnls. tilapia fillets
- 2 (or so) Tbls. olive oil
- 2 Tbls. lemon pepper seasoning
- 1 Tbls. garlic salt
- 3 Tbls. Fresh dill Chopped
- pinch of kosher salt
- juice of 1 Lemon

Direction

- Drizzle Olive Oil over fish.
- Season the fish with all the dry spices and Dill.
- Squeeze the juice of the lemon to cover the fish.
- Let marinate for 15 mins.
- Grill over med/high heat 6-8 mins per side until done (I use a fish grill basket that holds the fish in place while it cooks).

187. Lemon Parmesan Tilapia Recipe

Serving: 4 | Prep: | Cook: 15mins | Ready in:

Ingredients

- 2 egg whites
- 1/2 c grated parmesan cheese
- 2 Tb flour
- 2 Tb chopped parsley
- 1-1/2 tsp McCormick Cracked peppercorn Herb roasting Rub
- 1-1/2 tsp grated lemon zest
- 4 tilapia fillets (1-1/4 lbs)

Direction

- Beat egg whites in shallow dish; reserve. Combine parmesan, flour, parsley, peppercorn rub, and zest; spread on wax paper. Dip each fillet in egg, then in parmesan mixture, turning to coat completely.
- In large non-stick skillet, heat 2 tsp oil over med. heat. Add 2 fillets; cook turning once until opaque and lightly browned, about 3 mins. per side. Remove to serving platter. Repeat with remaining oil and fillets. If desired, garnish with lemon and rosemary.
- Note: For a change, serve halved fillets on a soft bun with tartar sauce, sliced tomato and lettuce leaves.

188. Lemon Rice With Crispy Salmon Recipe

Serving: 4 | Prep: | Cook: 35mins | Ready in:

Ingredients

- • 2 pouches (125 g each) Minute Rice Jasmine Rice
- • 3/4 cup (175 mL) frozen peas, thawed
- • 1/4 cup (60 mL) sliced green onion
- • 2 tbsp (30 mL) lemon juice
- • 4 skin-on salmon fillets (5 to 6 oz/140 to 170 g each)
- • 1/2 tsp (2 mL) salt
- • 1/4 tsp (1 mL) pepper
- • 2 tbsp (30 mL) canola oil
- • Lemon wedges

Direction

- Step 1: Cook rice according to package directions. Add peas during the last minute of cooking; stir in half of the green onion, and lemon juice.
- Step 2: Meanwhile, using a sharp knife, score skin side of salmon, slicing 1/2-inch (1 cm) across and about 1/4-inch (5 mm) deep; season all over with salt and pepper.
- Step 3: In large, heavy-bottom skillet, heat oil over medium-high heat; cook salmon skin side down for about 5 minutes or until skin is golden brown and crispy. Turn over; cook for 2 or 3 minutes or until fish is just cooked through and flakes easily with a fork. Serve with rice and lemon wedges. Sprinkle with remaining green onion.
- Nutrition Facts. Per 1/4 recipe: Calories 410, Fat 18g, Cholesterol 80mg, Sodium 450mg, Carbohydrate 29g, Fibre 2g, Sugars 2g, Protein 33g

189. Lemon Salmon Linguini Recipe

Serving: 4 | Prep: | Cook: 10mins | Ready in:

Ingredients

- 1Tbs. olive oil
- 1 pound salmon (boneless and skinless), cut into 2-inch chunks
- 1 tps. kosher salt
- 1/2 tps. fennel seed
- 1/4 tps. ground black pepper
- 1 1/2 cups thinly sliced red onion
- 1 1/2 cups cherry tomatoes, halved
- 1 cup ripe olives. halved
- 3/4 cup chicken broth
- 1/4 cup lemon juice
- 2 Tbs. Chopped dill
- 1 1/2 Tbs. minced lemon zest
- 1 quart (1 1/4 pound) cooked linguini pasta
- 6 ounces baby spinach

Direction

- Heat 1 Tbs. of olive oil in a large high-sided sauté pan over medium-high heat. Place salmon in pan, season with salt, fennel seed and pepper and cook for 4-5 minutes, turning occasionally, until golden and cooked through. Using a slotted spatula, transfer to a clean bowl and set aside.

- Heat remaining oil in pan, add onions and cook over medium heat for 3-4 minutes until tender. Stir in tomatoes, ripe olives, chicken broth, lemon juice, dill and lemon zest and bring to a boil.
- Mix in linguini and continue cooking until heated through. Gently toss with salmon and baby spinach and serve immediately.

190. Lemony Stuffed Flounder Fillets Recipe

Serving: 4 | Prep: | Cook: 30mins | Ready in:

Ingredients

- 1/3 C butter
- 1/3 C celery, chopped
- 2 Tbl onion, chopped
- 1 Tbl parsley
- 1 C herb seasoned stuffing
- 1 Tbl lemon juice
- 1 tsp lemon peel
- 1/4 tsp salt
- 1/4 tsp pepper
- 1 lb flounder or other white fish
- 1/3 C butter
- 1/2 tsp dill weed

Direction

- Preheat oven to 350.
- In a 1-qt. saucepan, melt butter and sauté celery and onion until tender.
- Stir in stuffing, parsley, lemon juice and peel, salt and pepper; set aside.
- Cut each fillet to make 8 halves; place 4 halves in an ungreased square baking dish or pan.
- Top each with 1/4 C of the stuffing and top with remaining halves.
- Melt 1/3 C butter; stir in dill weed.
- Pour dill butter over fillets.
- Bake in center of oven 20 to 30 minutes or until fish flakes.
- Spoon sauce over fish and return to oven for an additional 5 minutes.

191. Liffey Trout With Mushroom Sauce Recipe

Serving: 4 | Prep: | Cook: 25mins | Ready in:

Ingredients

- 4 small trout
- 6 Tbl flour
- salt and pepper
- 6 Tbl butter
- about 12 button mushrooms
- 1 C half cream and half milk
- 1 Tbl parsley

Direction

- Clean, wash and dry trout.
- Roll in 1/4 cup of the flour seasoned with salt and pepper.
- Fry fish in 1/4 cup of butter, drain and keep hot.
- Slice mushrooms and sauté in same pan used for the trout. Melt remaining butter in a small saucepan; stir in remaining flour.
- Add cream and milk and season to taste.
- Add mushrooms and reheat to serving temp.
- Garnish with parsley and serve sauce separately.
- 4 servings.

192. Light Alaskan Halibut Lasagna Diabetic Friendly Recipe

Serving: 8 | Prep: | Cook: 45mins | Ready in:

Ingredients

- Ingredients:
- 6 Tbs. light margarine
- 1 ½ pounds halibut steaks, bones removed and cut into 1-inch cubes
- 2 garlic cloves, minced
- ¾ tsp. Dried thyme
- 1/3 cup all-purpose flour
- ½ tsp. salt
- 1 ½ cups College Inn light + fat-free 50% less sodium chicken broth
- 1 cup heavy whipping cream
- 8 ounces Dreamfields low-calorie lasagna noodles, cooked and drained
- 2 cups (8-oz) shredded swiss cheese (Alpine Lace reduced-fat-sodium)
- Minced fresh parsley, optional

Direction

- Preheat oven to 350° F.
- In a large skillet over medium heat, melt 2 tablespoons of margarine. Add halibut, garlic and thyme. Cook until fish flakes easily with a fork, about 10 minutes. Remove and set aside. Add the remaining margarine to the skillet. Stir in flour and salt until smooth; cook and stir until golden brown. Gradually add broth and cream. Bring to a boil; cook and stir for 2 minutes or until thickened.
- In a greased 13-inch x 9-inch baking dish, layer half of the noodles, halibut, white sauce and cheese. Repeat layers. Cover and bake at 350° for 20 minutes. Uncover; bake longer or until bubbly. Let stand 15 minutes before serving. Sprinkle with parsley if desired. Yield: 8 servings.
- Serving size 1/8 of the lasagna
- Diabetic Friendly
- Nutritional Values: Calories per serving: 298, Fat: 10g, Cholesterol: 99mg, Sodium: 349mg, Carbohydrate: 24g Fiber: 2g, Protein: 30g

193. Mahi Mahi Tacos With Ginger Lime Dressing Recipe

Serving: 6 | Prep: | Cook: 10mins | Ready in:

Ingredients

- 1 tablespoon olive oil
- salt and pepper to taste
- 6 (3 ounce) fillets mahi mahi fillets
- 1/3 cup sour cream
- 1 tablespoon lime juice
- 1 teaspoon minced fresh ginger root
- 1/4 teaspoon ground cumin
- 1 dash cayenne pepper
- 1 large mango - peeled, seeded and diced
- 1 cup diced fresh pineapple
- 1 avocado - peeled, pitted and diced
- 1 jalapeno pepper, minced
- 6 (6 inch) flour tortillas, warmed
- 1 cup chopped fresh cilantro

Direction

- Heat the olive oil in a large skillet over medium-high heat.
- Season the mahi-mahi with salt and pepper.
- Cook the fillets in the hot oil until the fish is golden brown on each side, and no longer translucent in the center, about 3 minutes per side.
- Meanwhile, whisk together the sour cream, lime juice, ginger, cumin, cayenne pepper, salt and pepper to taste; set aside.
- Gently combine the mango, pineapple, avocado, and jalapeno in a bowl.
- To assemble, place a cooked mahi-mahi fillet into the center of a warmed tortilla.
- Place a scoop of the mango salsa onto the fish, then drizzle with the sour cream sauce, and finish with a generous pinch of chopped cilantro.

194. Maine Atlantic Top Stuffed Haddock Recipe

Serving: 4 | Prep: | Cook: 20mins | Ready in:

Ingredients

- 4 (6-8 oz) haddock or other white fish (firm)
- 4 oz canned crabmeat
- 4 oz can tiny shrimp
- 1 cup bread crumbs
- 2 tbsp thyme
- 1/3 cup olive oil
- 1/2 tsp lemon zest
- 1/2 stick butter melted**
- 2 tbsp olive oil**
- 1/4 cup white wine**
- salt & pepper

Direction

- In bowl:
- Toss bread crumbs, thyme, crabmeat, shrimp, oil (1/3 cup), zest, salt & pepper.
- Divide bread crumb mixture into 4 portions.
- Pat one portion on a piece of fish and continue with other 3 pieces of fish.
- Put in 9 x 13 pan. Bake at 350-degree oven.
- Mix together: **
- 1/2 stick melted butter
- 2 tbsp olive oil
- 1/4 cup white wine
- Pour over fish before baking.
- Bake 10-15 minutes or till fish flakes.

195. Maple Cured Cedar Planked Salmon Or Tofu With Chipotle Glaze And Blueberry Pico Recipe

Serving: 4 | Prep: | Cook: 15mins | Ready in:

Ingredients

- salmon fillet, Trimmed 1 Side (2.5-3#) [For Vegetarian - 1 brick of tofu, pressed of water]
- Serves: 1 salmon side 4-6 people
- Cedar Plank, big enough to fit the fillet, 1 each Clean and unfinished - soak in cool water for 3 hrs.)
- FOR THE BRINE
- water 1 qt
- sugar, Brown 1/2 c
- maple syrup 2 cups
- salt, Kosher 1 ½ cup
- sugar, granulated ½ cup
- rosemary or thyme, fresh 3 sprigs
- FOR THE CHIPOTLE glaze
- chipotle peppers 2-3 peppers with bit of sauce
- maple syrup 1 c
- FOR THE BLUEBERRY pico de gallo
- blueberries, fresh, washed 2 cups
- cucumber, seeded and diced 2 cups
- jalapeno, fresh minced 6 large
- onion, Red, diced small 1 large
- lime, juice and zest 2 large
- olive oil, Extra Virgin ½ cup
- cilantro, fresh, minced ½ bunch
- salt and FGBP to taste
- [I added about 1/8 cup of honey]

Direction

- Put together your Blueberry Pico de Gallo: Mix all ingredients and let sit at room temperature. After 3 hours adjust seasoning and serve. Serve room temperature.
- Yield: 4 cups
- Prepare the Brine for the salmon. Bring water, Brown Sugar, Maple Syrup, salt and granulated sugar to a boil to dissolve sugars;
- Add fresh herbs and chill brine. Once brine is chilli, add the side of salmon to and marinate for 1-hour. [Vegetarian notes: I just divided up the brine and put tofu in one container and salmon in the other]
- Remove from brine, discard brine and pat salmon dry. [No need to pat tofu dry]
- Preheat oven to 450-degrees, or grill to high heat
- Season fish with salt and pepper.

- Place fish on the plank, then place in a heated oven or on a charcoal grill for about 15 minutes, glaze with Chipotle & Maple Glaze, continue cooking to desired doneness
- Serve on plank garnished with fresh lemon wedges or transfer to a serving platter.

196. Maple Salmon Recipe

Serving: 4 | Prep: | Cook: 20mins | Ready in:

Ingredients

- 1/4 cup pure maple syrup
- 2 Tbs. soy sauce
- 1 clove garlic, minced
- 1/4 tsp. garlic salt
- 1/8 tsp. ground black pepper
- 1 pound salmon

Direction

- In a small bowl, mix the maple syrup, soy sauce, garlic, garlic salt and pepper.
- Place salmon in a shallow glass baking dish and coat with the maple syrup mixture. Cover the dish and marinade salmon in the refrigerator 30 minutes, turning once.
- Preheat oven to 400F (200C).
- Place the baking dish in the preheated oven and bake salmon uncovered 20 minutes or until it easily flakes with a fork.

197. Mediterranean Poached Bass Recipe

Serving: 4 | Prep: | Cook: 8mins | Ready in:

Ingredients

- 1 medium onion, chopped
- ½ red bell pepper, chopped
- 1 cubanelle pepper, seeded and diced
- 4 medium garlic cloves, minced
- 2 cups canned diced tomatoes
- ½ cup fish or vegetable broth
- 2 tbsp sliced green olives
- 2 tsp brined capers, drained
- 1 ½ pound sea bass, quartered

Direction

- Sauté onion and peppers 7 minutes in a large non-stick pan.
- Add garlic and cook 1 minute more.
- Stir tomatoes, broth, olives and capers into onion mixture and heat to simmer.
- Arrange fish in skillet. Cover and cook 8 to 10 minutes.
- To serve, remove fish to plates and spoon tomato and olive mixture over fish.

198. Mediterranean Tuna Steaks Recipe

Serving: 2 | Prep: | Cook: 8mins | Ready in:

Ingredients

- 2 tuna steaks, 6 ounces each, about 1 inch thick
- 2 teaspoons extra-virgin olive oil
- salt and pepper to taste
- 1 medium ripe tomato, diced fine
- 6 green olives, pitted and chopped
- 1 tablespoon scallions, chopped
- 2 teaspoons capers
- 1 clove garlic, mashed
- Pinch of dried whole oregano

Direction

- Rinse the tuna steaks under cold water and pat dry.
- Brush them with 1 teaspoon olive oil and season with salt and pepper.
- Preheat grill or broiler. Meanwhile, mix the remaining ingredients in a small bowl and set aside.

- Grill or broil the steaks on high heat, about 2-3 minutes per side or until desired doneness.
- Top the tuna steaks with the tomato-olive mixture.

199. Melissa DArabians Salmon Cakes Recipe

Serving: 4 | Prep: | Cook: 8mins | Ready in:

Ingredients

- 2 strips bacon, cooked until crispy, crumbled, bacon fat reserved
- 1/4 cup chopped onion
- 1 egg
- 1/2 cup mayonnaise
- 2 teaspoons Dijon mustard
- 1/2 teaspoon sugar
- 1/2 lemon, zested
- 1 (14-ounce) can wild salmon, checked for bones
- 1 baked or boiled russet potato, peeled, and fluffed with a fork
- 1/4 cup bread crumbs
- 2 tablespoons grated Parmesan
- Freshly ground black pepper
- 1/2 cup vegetable oil, divided

Direction

- Heat 1 tablespoon of the reserved bacon fat in a small sauté pan over low heat.
- Add the onions and cook until translucent.
- Set aside to cool.
- Mix the bacon, onion, egg, mayonnaise, mustard, sugar, and lemon zest in a bowl.
- Add the salmon and potato, mixing gently after each addition.
- Form the mixture into 12 small patties. (Use an ice cream scoop to make them uniform.)
- In a shallow dish, combine the bread crumbs, parmesan, and pepper, to taste.
- Coat the patties in the bread crumb topping.
- Heat 1/4 cup of the oil in a large sauté pan over medium heat.
- Cook the salmon cakes in batches until golden, about 3 to 4 minutes per side.
- Serve immediately

200. Mikes Favorite Fried Catfish Recipe

Serving: 4 | Prep: | Cook: 15mins | Ready in:

Ingredients

- 2 eggs
- ½ cup buttermilk
- 2 Tbsp hot sauce
- 1 cup corn meal
- 1 cup flour
- 2 tsp dried granulated onion
- 2 Tbsp dried granulated garlic
- ½ tsp ground cayenne pepper
- 1 tsp salt
- ½ tsp ground black pepper
- 4 lbs catfish filets
- oil for frying (corn oil or peanut oil works best)

Direction

- Place oil in a deep fryer and heat to 365.
- Mix eggs, buttermilk, and hot sauce in a bowl and beat well to make an egg wash.
- Mix cornmeal, flour granulated onion, granulated garlic, Cayenne pepper, salt and black pepper in a small casserole dish.
- Cut catfish filets into strips approx. 1 inch thickness.
- Place catfish strips in egg wash mixture and soak for 3-5 minutes.
- Remove catfish strips from egg wash and drain briefly.
- Roll wet catfish strips in flower mixture. Allow catfish strips to sit in flour for 1-2 minutes.
- Remove the catfish strips from flour, shake off excess flour and place into hot oil.

- Fry to a golden brown, turning often.
- Remove to drip pan or paper towels to drain grease.
- Season to taste and serve with tartar sauce, hushpuppies and slaw.
- It's a good idea to ice down the beers before you start this recipe so they're good and cold at serving time!

201. Miso Salmon With Sake Butter Recipe

Serving: 4 | Prep: | Cook: 30mins | Ready in:

Ingredients

- 1/4 cup brown sugar, packed
- 2 tablespoons low sodium soy sauce
- 2 tablespoons hot water
- 2 tablespoons miso (soybean paste)
- 4 (6 ounce) salmon fillets (about 1 inch thick)
- cooking spray
- 1 tablespoon fresh chives, chopped
- cooked rice
- sake butter ingredients
- 2 tablespoons peeled and julienned ginger
- 1 tablespoon minced shallots
- 1 tablespoon unsalted butter
- 1/2 cup plus 1 teaspoon quality sake (Momokawa)
- 1 tablespoon heavy cream
- 1/2 cup (1 stick) cold unsalted butter, cut into large dice
- 1/2 teaspoons fresh lime juice
- Kosher salt

Direction

- Preheat broiler.
- Combine first 4 ingredients, stirring with a whisk.
- Arrange fish in a shallow baking dish coated with cooking spray.
- Spoon miso mixture evenly over fish.
- Broil 10 minutes or until fish flakes easily when tested with a fork, basting twice with miso mixture.
- Sprinkle with chives.
- Sake Butter
- In a small saucepan over medium-high heat, sweat the ginger and shallots in the one tablespoon butter for two to three minutes.
- Add 1/2 cup of the sake, bring to a boil, and reduce by two-thirds, about three minutes.
- Add the heavy cream, bring to a boil, and reduce by half, about two minutes.
- Add the pieces of cold butter to the sauce, bit by bit, whisking constantly over medium-high heat. The butter will emulsify, creating a thick creamy sauce.
- Once all the butter has been incorporated, remove the pan from the heat. Whisk in the remaining one teaspoon sake and the lime juice.
- Season to taste with salt.
- Place Sake butter on plate, top with a bed of rice, place salmon on top of rice.

202. Miso Marinated Salmon With Cucumber Daikon Relish Recipe

Serving: 6 | Prep: | Cook: 15mins | Ready in:

Ingredients

- 1/4 cup white miso (fermented soybean paste)
- 1/4 cup mirin (sweet Japanese rice wine)
- 2 tablespoons unseasoned rice vinegar
- 2 tablespoons minced green onions
- 1 1/2 tablespoons minced fresh ginger
- 2 teaspoons oriental sesame oil
- 6 6-ounce Alaskan salmon fillets, with skin
- Nonstick vegetable oil spray
- ~~~~
- cucumber-Daikon Relish:
- 2 English hothouse cucumbers, peeled, halved, seeded, cut crosswise into 1/4-inch-thick slices

- 2 teaspoons sea salt
- 8 ounces daikon (Japanese white radish), peeled, cut into 2x1/4-inch sticks
- 2/3 cup unseasoned rice vinegar
- 2/3 cup sugar
- 1 tablespoon minced fresh ginger
- 1/8 teaspoon cayenne pepper
- ~~~~
- 1 1/2 teaspoons sesame seeds, toasted
- 1/2 cup radish sprouts
- 1/2 8x8-inch sheet dried nori,* cut with scissors into matchstick-size strips

Direction

- Make Cucumber-Daikon Relish:
- Toss cucumbers with sea salt in colander. Place colander over bowl and let stand 15 minutes. Rinse cucumbers. Drain and pat dry with paper towels.
- Place radish sticks in medium bowl. Cover with water. Soak 15 minutes. Drain and pat dry with paper towels.
- Stir vinegar and next 3 ingredients in large bowl to blend. Add cucumbers and radish; toss to coat. Cover and chill at least 30 minutes and up to 2 hours.
- ~~~~
- Whisk first 6 ingredients in 13x9x2-inch glass baking dish to blend for marinade. Add salmon; turn to coat. Cover and chill at least 30 minutes and up to 2 hours.
- Preheat broiler. Line heavy large baking sheet with foil; spray with non-stick spray.
- Remove salmon fillets from miso marinade; using rubber spatula, scrape off excess marinade. Arrange salmon, skin side up, on prepared baking sheet.
- Broil 5 to 6 inches from heat source until skin is crisp, about 2 minutes. Using metal spatula, turn salmon over. Broil until salmon is just cooked through and golden brown on top, about 4 minutes.
- Transfer salmon to plates, skin side down. Spoon Cucumber Relish over. Sprinkle with sesame seeds, then sprouts and nori. Serve immediately.

203. Mississippi Delta Fried Catfish Recipe

Serving: 4 | Prep: | Cook: 15mins | Ready in:

Ingredients

- 3/4 cup yellow cornmeal
- 1/4 cup selfrising flour (or plain flour and 1/4 tsp baking powder)
- 1/2 tsp salt
- 1/2 tsp black pepper
- 1 tsp garlic powder or grandulated
- 1/2 tsp cayenne pepper (optional)
- 2 lbs Catfish filets
- Good quality vegetable or peanut oil for deep frying.
- Note(1) Allow two or three 5 to 7 oz fillets per person.
- Note: (2) if not using cayenne pepper, crack a little black pepper on filets before dredging.

Direction

- Mix dry ingredients. Fish should be moist to capture batter. Do not towel dry. Coat fish evenly and drop in hot oil (360 degrees) Fish will turn golden and float to top when done. Do not overcrowd. Immediately place on absorbent paper. A brown grocery bag topped with paper towels works great.

204. Moist Baked Tilapia Recipe

Serving: 6 | Prep: | Cook: 20mins | Ready in:

Ingredients

- 6 Tilapia filets (I buy the individually frozen ones from Costco, they also sell it fresh at times)
- ranch dressing (I use Hidden Valley Light bottled)
- bacon (I use Hormel Real Crumbled bacon in the bag - convenient and less fat and hassle)
- 1/4 cup chopped sweet onion (or I have used red, green or yellow - whatever you have)
- Parmesan (or whatever cheese your like) That's what this recipe is all about - convenience!

Direction

- Preheat oven to 375°F.
- Place Tilapia fillets in greased 9x13 (or whatever works for you).
- Spread ranch dressing on each one - as thin or thick as you like.
- Sprinkle with bacon bits as much as you like.
- Sprinkle with onion.
- Top with the cheese (I wait until last 5 minutes of cooking - but you choose when).
- Bake in oven for 15 - 20 minutes max - Don't want them dry.
- You can use them frozen and cook 30 mins at 375° and it works just as well.

205. Mojo Bass Recipe

Serving: 4 | Prep: | Cook: 9mins | Ready in:

Ingredients

- 1 tablespoon fresh orange juice
- 1 tablespoon fresh lime juice
- 1 teaspoon ground coriander
- 1 teaspoon bottled minced garlic
- 1 teaspoon olive oil
- 1/2 teaspoon ground cumin
- 4 (6-ounce) striped bass fillets (about 1 inch thick)
- cooking spray
- 2 tablespoons chopped fresh mint

Direction

- Preheat broiler.
- Combine first 6 ingredients, stirring with a whisk.
- Arrange fish, skin side down, on a foil-lined baking sheet coated with cooking spray. Brush half of orange juice mixture over fish; broil 4 minutes. Brush with remaining orange juice mixture; broil 4 minutes or until fish flakes easily when tested with a fork. Sprinkle with mint.

206. Moroccan Grilled Salmon Recipe

Serving: 4 | Prep: | Cook: 15mins | Ready in:

Ingredients

- 1/2 cup plain yogurt
- juice of 1 lemon, plus lemon wedges for garnish
- 1 tablespoon extra-virgin olive oil, plus more for the grill
- 2 to 3 cloves garlic, smashed
- 1 1/2 teaspoons ground coriander
- 1 1/2 teaspoons ground cumin
- kosher salt and freshly ground pepper
- 4 6-ounce skinless center-cut salmon fillets
- 1/4 cup chopped fresh cilantro or parsley, for garnish

Direction

- Stir together the yogurt, lemon juice, olive oil, garlic, coriander, cumin, 1/4 teaspoon salt, and pepper to taste in a small bowl. Pour half of the sauce into a large resealable plastic bag; cover and refrigerate the remaining sauce. Add the salmon to the bag and turn to coat with the marinade. Refrigerate for 20 to 30 minutes, turning the bag over once.
- Preheat a grill to medium-high. Remove the salmon from the marinade and blot off excess

yogurt with paper towels. Lightly oil the grill and add the salmon; cook, turning once, until browned on the outside and opaque in the center, 4 to 6 minutes per side, depending on the thickness. Serve with the reserved yogurt sauce and garnish with the herbs and lemon wedges.

207. New Bedford Flounder Roll Ups Recipe

Serving: 6 | Prep: | Cook: 25mins | Ready in:

Ingredients

- 6 large flounder fillets
- 4 strips of bacon
- ¼ C melted butter
- 3 C cornbread crumbs
- ¼ tsp chervil
- ¼ tsp dried tarragon leaves
- hot water
- butter

Direction

- Cook bacon until crisp; drain on paper towels
- Measure ¼ C bacon drippings and add to melted butter
- Combine cornbread crumbs, bacon, herbs and butter mixture; mix well
- Add enough hot water to make stuffing as moist as desired
- Place a spoonful of stuffing on each fillet; roll up firmly
- Place seam side down in a sprayed baking dish; dot generously with butter
- Bake at 375 for 25 minutes or until fish flakes easily with a fork

208. Nutty Hot Cod Fillets Recipe

Serving: 6 | Prep: | Cook: 20mins | Ready in:

Ingredients

- 2 1/4 lbs of cod fillets, fairly thick
- 1/2 to 3/4 cup of mayonnaise, good quality
- 1/2 to 3/4 cup of chopped pecans (ummmm, don't bother toasting in butter) and only if you are completely patient, pistachios (oh, the shelling!)
- 2 tablespoons of horseradish, scant amount
- 1/4 teaspoon of turmeric
- 1/4 teaspoon of salt
- olive oil or butter (use those saved butter wrappers in your freezer)

Direction

- Preheat oven to 400 degrees.
- Double wrap a cookie sheet with foil. Lightly oil with a mild flavored oil or coat with a scant amount of butter.
- Place cod fillets on prepped pan.
- Mix mayonnaise, nuts, horseradish, and turmeric, and salt. Spread over the fish.
- Bake in hot oven for twenty minutes, until golden brown on top and bubbly. Serve with lemon wedges and cracked black pepper.

209. OLIVE DIPPER N SOLE Recipe

Serving: 4 | Prep: | Cook: 5mins | Ready in:

Ingredients

- Olive Cream Sauce:
- 1/4 cup. plain yogurt
- 1/4 cup. mayonaise
- 1/2 tsp. grated lime zest
- 2 tsp. lime juice
- 1 tsp olive juice

- 2 tbsp. minced green olives
- 1 tbsp. chopped mixed fresh herbs (such as dill, oregano, thyme)
- 1 1/2 lbs.sole
- flour for dusting
- vegetable oil, for deep frying
- salt and pepper to taste
- Batter:
- 3/4 cup flour
- 1/4 cup grated parmesan cheese
- 1 tsp. baking soda
- 1 egg, separated
- 2/3 cup buttermilk
- 1/2 cup water
- salt & pepper to taste

Direction

- To make the Cream Sauce:
- Mix yogurt, mayonnaise, lime zest, lime & olive juice, olives, and herbs together.
- Place in the fridge to chill.
- To make the batter:
- Mix the flour, Parmesan, soda and a pinch of salt.
- Whisk in the egg yolk and buttermilk in to the batter to make it thick, but smooth.
- Gradually whisk in the water.
- Season with salt and pepper.
- Whisk the egg white until stiff in a separate bowl.
- Gently fold it into the batter until just blended.
- Skin the fish and cut it into strips.
- Place the flour in a large shallow plate and season it with salt and pepper.
- Dredge the fish in the seasoned flour, shaking off any excess.
- Heat a deep fryer to about 350F. Dip the floured fish into batter, then drop gently into the hot oil.
- Cook fish for about 4-5 minutes, turning once.
- Cook in batches to prevent the oil from cooling down and to keep the strips from sticking to each other.
- When the batter is golden brown, and crisp, remove the fish and drain on paper towels.
- Serve hot, accompanied by the Olive Cream Sauce.

210. Old World Recipe Fish In Tomato Sauce Recipe

Serving: 6 | Prep: | Cook: 60mins | Ready in:

Ingredients

- 2 lbs white firm fleshed fish, such as carp, cod, hake, catfish, etc... Use fillets or steaks cut in halves, with back bone removed.
- 4 large onions, finely chopped
- 1 small can tomato paste
- 1/2 cup flour
- salt, pepper, sugar to taste
- allspice whole corns
- bay leaves
- coriander seed
- cooking oil
- butter

Direction

- Cut fish into serving pieces, about 1-1/2 x 4 inches each. Leave the skin on if desire
- Add about 1 tbsp. salt and 1/2 tbsp. pepper to flour and mix well
- Heat 4-5 tbsp. cooking oil in a skillet, add 1 tbsp. butter
- Drench each fish piece in flour mix and fry on all sides until pleasantly browned
- Remove fish from the skillet and place in a saucepan, Dutch oven or medium pot
- Melt 1-2 tbsp. butter in another skillet and sauté onions until golden-brown and most of the liquid is evaporated
- Add 1 tbsp. of the drenching flour mix to the onions and cook, constantly stirring for another minute or so
- Stir in 2-3 cups of water, 2 tbsp. sugar, salt and pepper to taste.
- Add coriander, whole spice, and mix well

- Add tomato paste and stir until all is smooth and tomato paste is dissolved.
- Adjust the flavor if necessary to result into punchy sweet and sour sauce
- Pour tomato sauce over the fish, bring to boil
- Simmer over very low flame for about 45 minutes
- Add 3-4 bay leaves and simmer for another 3-4 minutes.
- -
- Add fresh chopped parsley before serving
- Serve hot over mashed potatoes, or cold.

211. One Dish Poached Halibut And Vegetables Recipe

Serving: 4 | Prep: | Cook: 12mins | Ready in:

Ingredients

- 2 cups thinly sliced fennel bulb (about 6 ounces)
- 2 cups organic vegetable broth (such as Swanson Certified Organic)
- 1 (20-ounce) package refrigerated red potato wedges (such as Simply potatoes)
- 8 ounces baby carrots
- 4 (6-ounce) halibut fillets
- 1/2 teaspoon paprika
- 1/8 teaspoon salt
- 1/8 teaspoon freshly ground black pepper
- 1/2 teaspoon chopped fresh thyme
- 4 lemon wedges

Direction

- Combine first 4 ingredients in a large non-stick skillet; bring to a boil. Cover, reduce heat, and simmer 4 minutes.
- Sprinkle one side of fish with paprika, salt, and pepper. Add fish, seasoning side up, and thyme to pan; bring to a boil. Cover, reduce heat, and simmer 6 minutes or until fish flakes easily when tested with a fork or until desired degree of doneness. Serve with lemon wedges.

212. Orange And Fennel Glazed Salmon Recipe

Serving: 4 | Prep: | Cook: 10mins | Ready in:

Ingredients

- 4 six ounce portions of one inch thick salmon fillets
- 1/2 tsp of salt and 1/2 tsp of black pepper
- 2 teaspoons of grated orange rind
- equal portions of fresh rosemary leaves and fennel seeds
- 1/2 cup of fresh orange juice
- cooking spray

Direction

- Combine orange juice, orange rind and crushed rosemary leaves and fennel seeds.
- I use a mortar and pestle for the rosemary and fennel.
- Put fish and marinade in a large resealable plastic bag.
- Refrigerate 20 minutes. Turning at least once.
- Meanwhile preheat broiler.
- Remove fish from marinade, reserving the marinade.
- Place fish skin side down on a broiler pan well coated with non-stick cooking spray.
- Season liberally with salt and pepper.
- Broil about 10 minutes.
- Bring reserved marinade to a boil in a small sauce pan, reduce heat and simmer while the salmon cooks.
- Serve the sauce with the finished salmon.
- I like peas with this dish especially the braised peas with lettuce and a mushroom rice pilaf.

213. Orange And Ginger Halibut Steaks Recipe

Serving: 4 | Prep: | Cook: 6mins | Ready in:

Ingredients

- juice of 1 orange
- 2 T brown sugar
- 1" piece of fresh ginger (peeled and minced)
- 1 T orange marmalade
- 5 cloves garlic minced
- 4 halibut steaks, about 6oz each
- 2 T olive oil
- 1 ½ T light soy sauce

Direction

- Combine the orange juice, sugar, ginger, marmalade and garlic in a blender, puree. Pour into a shallow casserole or baking dish; add halibut. Set aside to let marinate about 20 minutes.
- Drain, reserving marinade. Heat oil in a large skillet over medium-high heat. Add the halibut steaks; cook until the fish browns around the edges, about 5 minutes. Turn; lower heat to medium. Cook until the fish flakes easily, about 4 minutes. Transfer to a platter. Add the reserved marinade to the skillet. Raise the heat to medium-high. Add the soy sauce; heat to a boil. Cook until mixture thickens, about 1 ½ minutes.

214. Orange Glazed Salmon Fillets With Rosemary Recipe

Serving: 4 | Prep: | Cook: 10mins | Ready in:

Ingredients

- 4 (6-ounce) salmon fillets (1 inch thick)
- 1/2 tsp kosher salt
- 1/4 tsp freshly ground black pepper
- cooking spray
- 2 Tbs minced shallots
- 1/4 cup dry white wine
- 1/2 tsp chopped fresh rosemary
- 3/4 cup fresh orange juice (about 2 oranges)*
- 1 Tbs maple syrup
- *I used juice from a carton and thought it tasted fine.

Direction

- Sprinkle fillets evenly with salt and pepper. Heat a large nonstick skillet over medium-high heat. Coat pan with cooking spray. Add fillets; cook 2 minutes on each side or until fish flakes easily when tested with a fork or until desired degree of doneness. Remove from pan.
- Recoat pan with cooking spray. Add shallots; sauté 30 seconds. Stir in wine and rosemary; cook 30 seconds or until liquid almost evaporates. Add juice and syrup; bring to a boil, and cook 1 minute. Return fillets to pan; cook 1 minute on each side or until thoroughly heated.

215. Oriental Salmon Recipe

Serving: 2 | Prep: | Cook: 20mins | Ready in:

Ingredients

- 2 skinless salmon fillets
- 2 tablespoons sesame oil
- 2 tablespoons black sesame seeds
- 1 teaspoon salt
- 2 tablespoons minced garlic
- 2 tablespoons freshly minced ginger
- 1/2 cup sugar
- 1 cup soy sauce
- 2 tablespoons cornstarch mixed with 2 tablespoons water
- 1-1/2 cups fresh Asian vegetables of your choice
- 1-1/2 tablespoons vegetable oil to sauté vegetables
- Steamed white rice

Direction

- Preheat oven to 450.
- Season fillets by coating with 1 tablespoon sesame oil then the sesame seeds.
- Add salt to taste.
- Set in a baking pan or cookie sheet with sides and bake in preheated oven for 15 minutes.
- While fish is baking make sauce by combining garlic, ginger, sugar, remaining 1 tablespoon sesame oil and the soy sauce in a small saucepan.
- Bring to a boil then reduce heat to a simmer and cook 5 minutes.
- In small bowl mix cornstarch and water until smooth.
- Slowly add some of the mixture to the sauce and cook until thick enough to coat the back of a spoon.
- Add cornstarch mixture as needed.
- Sauté vegetables in the vegetable oil in a covered sauté pan until tender.
- When vegetables are tender add sauce and gently mix then spoon vegetables over baked fillets and serve immediately over steamed rice.

216. Oven Fried Catfish That Tastes Like Real Fried Recipe

Serving: 6 | Prep: | Cook: 20mins | Ready in:

Ingredients

- catfish fillets (5-7 oz) or other fish fillets
- cornmeal (Stoneground or course ground preferred)
- granulated garlic
- salt and black pepper

Direction

- Season cornmeal with granulated garlic, salt and pepper to taste.
- Fish should be slightly damp, but not wet.
- Dredge fish in cornmeal and press meal into fish.
- Place on greased wire rack and place on baking pan
- Bake at 375 until golden brown and fish flakes, about 20 minutes.
- Note: The recipe for real Fried Catfish is posted on my page. This recipe was requested by a cooking friend who does not eat fried foods. Enjoy!
- Note: Farm-raised catfish has a white, mild and delicate flavor due to the fact that it is raised in special ponds and fed a diet of grains. The entire pond is netted and kept alive until processing time. From live to frozen fillets takes just minutes. Thus, no fishy taste.

217. Oven Slow Cook Salmon Recipe

Serving: 4 | Prep: | Cook: 30mins | Ready in:

Ingredients

- 4 (8 ounce) salmon fillets
- 1-2 tablespoons vegetable oil
- 3 navel oranges, cut into 1/4 inch slices
- 2 large onions, thinly sliced
- 1 large or 2 small fresh fennel bulbs, thinly sliced
- 3-4 sprigs fresh tarragon
- salt and pepper to taste
- Assorted garnishes such as crème fraiche, sliced oranges or fresh herbs

Direction

- Preheat to 250F. Lightly brush salmon with oil and season with salt and pepper. Let sit at room temperature for about 20 minutes.
- Grab a baking pan big enough to hold all fillets in single layer. Make a bed on the pan by layering the onions, fennel and two of the sliced oranges. Place the salmon fillets on the bed and tuck in the tarragon sprigs.

- Bake for 30 minutes. (If you're cooking more than 4 fillets, just add another 2 minutes per additional filet.) To test for doneness, stick a sharp paring knife in, if it goes in and out, it's done.
- Top with whatever finishing herbs, spices or ingredients you've chosen. After cooking, the salmon is going to look almost exactly the same as when you first put it in. Don't worry, after 30 minutes in the oven it will be cooked.
- Dress up your salmon however you like.

218. Pan Seared King Salmon And Diver Scallop With Sauce Piperade And A Horseradish Emulsion Recipe

Serving: 8 | Prep: | Cook: 6mins | Ready in:

Ingredients

- For the Piperade:
- 1 1/2 oz. spanish olive Oil
- 1 sweet onion, finely diced
- 1 Tbsp. garlic, finely minced
- 1 fennel bulb, finely diced
- 1 red bell pepper, finely diced
- 4-5 Vine Ripened tomatoes, seeds removed and finely diced
- 1 serrano chili, roasted and finely diced
- Sherry vinegar, to taste
- smoked paprika, to taste
- kosher salt, to taste
- Finely minced chives
- For the horseradish Emulsion:
- 2 cups water
- 2/3 cup prepared horseradish
- 4 oz. unsalted butter
- kosher salt to taste
- 2 tsp. Lecithin
- For the Seafood:
- 8 ea., 5 oz. fillets, fresh King salmon, rolled into a roulade and held with a wooden skewer to hold its shape (optional)
- 8 ea., U-10 Diver scallops, scored on one side
- kosher salt
- cooking oil

Direction

- For the Piperade:
- Pre-heat oven to 400 degrees F. Lightly coat the serrano chili with some oil, place on a pan, and roast until all sides are charred and the skin is peeling away. This can also be done over a grill or open flame. Place the chili in a bowl and cover with plastic wrap for 5 minutes so that the steam will help the skin pull away. When cool, peel, remove seeds, and finely dice. Meanwhile, heat the olive oil in a large sauté pan on medium high. Add the onion and garlic, and cook until the onion is translucent and tender, but do not brown. Add the fennel and bell pepper, and cook until tender. Add the tomatoes and serrano chili, and cook until the tomatoes are soft but still have a little shape. Season to taste with the sherry vinegar, smoked paprika, and kosher salt. Reserve and re-heat when needed. Add chives just before plating.
- For the Horseradish Emulsion:
- Heat the water and butter until the butter is dissolved and the mixture is hot. Whisk in the horseradish, lecithin, and a fair amount of salt. Aerate the liquid with an immersion blender to form the foam. Taste the foam and adjust seasoning. Add more horseradish and salt if needed, add butter to balance if too bitter. The foam should be intensely flavored or else it won't stand up against the piperade. Keep warm, and heat to 120-130 degrees F to foam.
- For the Seafood:
- Pre-heat oven to 400 degrees F. Heat oil on high. Season the salmon and scallop with kosher salt. Sear both seafoods on one side (add scallop scored side down) until golden brown. Turn over, briefly sear on bottom and finish in oven until medium rare doneness, about 3 minutes. Serve with the piperade sauce and horseradish emulsion.

219. Pan Seared Salmon And Scallops Umeboshi And Port Wine Reduction Sauce Plum Wine Emulsion Recipe

Serving: 6 | Prep: | Cook: 30mins | Ready in:

Ingredients

- 6 ea., 5 oz. Fresh King salmon fillets
- 12 ea., Atlantic Diver scallops, scored one one side and cleaned
- 1/2 bottle ruby port
- 1/3 lb. unsalted butter, cut into small cubes
- 2 tsp. Umeboshi paste
- 1 cup Japanese plum wine
- 1/4 cup Elderflower (sub. mirin or simple syrup)
- 2 tsp. Lecithin
- kosher salt to taste
- 1-2 tsp. Togarashi Shichimi
- canola oil

Direction

- In a sauce pan, reduce the port until the consistency of maple syrup. Remove from heat and whisk in the butter, a few cubes at a time until emulsified. Return to heat if the sauce gets cold, but do not boil. Whisk in the umeboshi paste and check for seasoning. Add more paste if needed. Reserve and keep warm.
- In a separate sauce pan, bring the plum wine to a boil and simmer for 3-4 minutes to cook off some of the alcohol and to take off the "bite" from it. Remove from heat and add the butter, elderflower, and lecithin. Season to taste and foam with an immersion blender (you'll need a good amount of salt to bring out the flavors).
- Heat enough oil in two large sauté pans on high until smoking. Score the skin side of the salmon and season with salt. Add skin side down and press down gently so that it sears evenly. Cook on high for 1 minute, then reduce heat to medium. Cook until the skin is golden brown and crispy, then flip and cook until medium doneness.
- Heat enough oil in two large sauté pans on high until smoking. Season the scallops with salt, and add the scored side down while pressing gently on each scallop so that it sears evenly. Cook until golden brown on each side, and until medium doneness.
- Serve the salmon and scallops with the two sauces layered, and a sprinkling of the togarashi on top.

220. Pan Seared Salmon With A Ginger Scallion Cilantro Pesto Recipe

Serving: 8 | Prep: | Cook: 15mins | Ready in:

Ingredients

- For the salmon:
- 8 ea., 7-8 oz. salmon filets
- 6 Tbsp. olive oil
- kosher salt
- fresh cracked pepper
- For the Pesto:
- 3/4 to 1 c. macadamia nut oil
- 1 c. loosely packed fresh cilantro leaves (thin stems are ok)
- 1/2 c. chopped scallions
- 1/2 c. Unsalted macadamia nuts
- 3 Tbsp. fresh ginger, chopped
- 1 Tbsp. fresh garlic, chopped
- juice of 1 lemon + the zest
- kosher salt to taste

Direction

- In a food processor or blender, combine all of the ingredients for the pesto and blend until you get a medium-thick pesto consistency. Add more oil as needed. Season to taste with kosher salt and reserve.

- Heat 3 Tbsp. of oil in two large sauté pans until lightly smoking. Season both sides of the salmon with kosher salt and pepper, carefully lay the salmon into the pans, skins side down. Cook the salmon until about medium doneness, about 3-4 minutes per side. Serve with the pesto drizzled on top and around the salmon.

221. Pan Seared Scarlet Red Snapper Crispy Polenta With Roasted Shallot Vinaigrette Recipe

Serving: 2 | Prep: | Cook: 10mins | Ready in:

Ingredients

- For the Crispy polenta
- 1 pre cooked polenta loaf sliced into ¾ inch rounds
- 4 tablespoons olive oil
- 2 tablespoons butter
- cilantro for garnish
- parsley for garnish
- lemon wedges
- cajun seasoning
- roasted shallot Vinaigrette:
- 4 shallots, peeled
- 1 cup olive oil
- 3 tablespoons balsamic vinegar
- 2 tablespoons chopped fresh chives
- salt and pepper
- For the red Snapper:
- 2 one inches of fresh Snapper about 6 oz each
- cajun seasoning
- 6 tablespoons of olive oil infused with shallots

Direction

- To make the crispy polenta, cut slices polenta loaf and sauté them in oil and butter.
- In a skillet, heat half the oil and half the butter. When the butter melts, fry the polenta slices without crowding over medium high heat, turning often, until they are golden brown and crisp. Fry the remaining slices in the same way.
- Remove from pan and lightly sprinkle with Cajun seasoning.
- Place in a warm oven.
- Directions for Vinaigrette:
- To prepare the vinaigrette: Place the shallots and 3/4 cup of the olive oil in a small ovenproof pan and cover tightly. Bake at 350 degrees for 50 to 60 minutes, or until the shallots are soft. Let the shallots cool in the olive oil, and then remove, reserving the oil. Julienne the shallots and put them in a bowl. Add the balsamic vinegar and slowly whisk in the reserved olive oil. Add the chopped chives and season to taste with salt and pepper.
- Directions for the Scarlet red Snapper:
- Sprinkle some Cajun seasoning on Snapper.
- In a fry pan, heat the oil until it shimmers.
- Add the Snapper skin side down and fry until it is browned and releases from the pan, about 4 minutes.
- Lower heat to medium, turn over and cook until browned remove and let rest.
- In a plate, spread some vinaigrette with shallots on each plate.
- Add the Crispy Polenta then top with the Snapper.
- Squeeze some fresh lemon on fish if desired.
- Top fish with more vinaigrette and garnish with parsley.
- Add the Salsa Verde on the side.
- Add tomato salsa and garnish with cilantro.
- Garnish with fresh lemon wedges and parsley.

222. Pan Seared White Wine Salmon Recipe

Serving: 4 | Prep: | Cook: 5mins | Ready in:

Ingredients

- 1 to 1 1/2 lbs fresh salmon
- 1/4 tsp salt
- 1/2 tsp course black pepper
- 1/2 tsp paprika
- 1/2 tsp basil
- 1/4 tsp dill weed
- 3/4 stick butter
- 1 Tblsp lemon juice
- 1/4 cup white wine
- 2 Tblsp olive oil
- (optinal for a sweeter tasting salmon, also add brown sugar to taste in sauce)

Direction

- Heat olive oil in skillet until almost smoking. Sprinkle salt and pepper on fillets and sear on both sides for 2 to 3 minutes until darkened.
- Melt butter in small sauce pan and add wine, lemon juice and remaining dry spices. Remove salmon from skillet and place on a plate and pour sauce over all. Enjoy!!
- This can also be done on the grill by coating the fillets with olive oil, sprinkling dry ingredients on fillets while on grill and use butter, wine and dry ingredients for sauce too. Takes 2 to 3 minutes per side.

223. Pan Seared Swordfish Steaks With Shallot Caper And Balsamic Sauce Recipe

Serving: 2 | Prep: | Cook: 15mins | Ready in:

Ingredients

- two 1-inch-thick swordfish steaks, each about 6 ounces
- 1 tablespoon unsalted butter
- 1/2 tablespoon olive oil
- 3 shallots, sliced thin
- 1/4 cup dry white wine
- 2 tablespoons balsamic vinegar
- 1 tablespoon drained capers, chopped
- 1 tablespoon water
- 1 tablespoon chopped fresh parsley leaves (wash and dry before chopping)

Direction

- Pat swordfish dry and season with salt and pepper. In a heavy skillet heat butter and oil over moderately high heat until foam subsides and sauté shallots with salt to taste, stirring, 1 minute.
- Push shallots to side of skillet. Add swordfish and sauté until golden, about 3 minutes.
- Turn fish over and add wine, vinegar, capers, and water. Simmer mixture 3 minutes, or until fish is just cooked through.
- Transfer fish to 2 plates and stir parsley into sauce. Spoon sauce over fish.

224. Pan Seared Tuna With Ginger Shiitake Cream Sauce Recipe

Serving: 6 | Prep: | Cook: 15mins | Ready in:

Ingredients

- 6 6-ounce tuna steaks, each about 1 inch thick
- 2 tablespoons peanut oil
- 3 tablespoons butter
- 1/3 cup thinly sliced green onions
- 1/4 cup chopped cilantro
- 2 tablespoons finely chopped peeled fresh ginger
- 4 garlic cloves, chopped
- 8 ounces fresh shiitake mushrooms, stemmed, caps sliced
- 6 tablespoons soy sauce
- 1 1/2 cups whipping cream
- 3 tablespoons fresh lime juice
- Lime wedges (optional)
- Fresh cilantro sprigs (optional)

Direction

- Preheat oven to 200°F. Sprinkle 1 side of tuna steaks with pepper. Heat 2 tablespoons oil in heavy large skillet over high heat. Place tuna steaks, pepper side down, in hot oil and sear 2 minutes. Turn tuna over and continue cooking to desired doneness, about 2 minutes for rare. Transfer tuna to rimmed baking sheet; keep warm in oven.
- Add butter, sliced green onions, cilantro, ginger and chopped garlic to same skillet and sauté until fragrant, about 30 seconds. Mix in mushrooms and soy sauce and simmer 30 seconds. Add whipping cream and simmer until sauce lightly coats back of spoon, about 3 minutes. Stir in lime juice. Spoon sauce onto plates; arrange tuna atop sauce. Garnish with lime wedges and cilantro sprigs, if desired.

225. Pan Fried Salmon Burgers With Cabbage Slaw And Avocado Aioli Recipe

Serving: 6 | Prep: | Cook: 20mins | Ready in:

Ingredients

- 1 1/2 pounds skinless center-cut salmon fillet, finely chopped
- 1/2 cup mayonnaise
- 2 tablespoons Asian fish sauce
- 2 tablespoons sambal oelek (see Note) or hot sauce
- 2 garlic cloves, minced
- 1 medium shallot, minced
- 1 tablespoon minced fresh ginger
- 1/2 teaspoon finely grated lemon zest
- 1/2 cup plus 2 tablespoons chopped cilantro
- 1/2 cup plus 1 tablespoon chopped mint
- kosher salt and freshly ground pepper
- 1 1/2 cups Japanese panko or plain dry bread crumbs
- 2 tablespoons fresh lemon juice
- 2 tablespoons fresh lime juice
- 2 tablespoons unseasoned rice vinegar
- 1 teaspoon sugar
- 1/2 small green cabbage, shredded
- 1 small cucumber – peeled, halved lengthwise, seeded and julienned
- 1 small red onion, thinly sliced
- 1 small red bell pepper, thinly sliced
- 1/4 cup sesame seeds
- 1/4 cup vegetable oil
- avocado Aioli, for serving
- 6 onion rolls, split and toasted

Direction

- In a food processor, pulse the chopped salmon about 10 times, or until minced. Scrape the salmon into a bowl. Mix the mayonnaise with the fish sauce, sambal oelek, garlic, shallot, ginger, lemon zest, 2 tablespoons of the cilantro, 1 tablespoon of the mint, 1 teaspoon of salt and 1/2 teaspoon of pepper. Add the mixture to the salmon along with 1 cup of the panko. Fold the salmon mixture together with a rubber spatula. With lightly oiled hands, pat the mixture into 6 burgers. Cover with plastic wrap and refrigerate for 2 hours.
- Meanwhile, in a large bowl, combine the lemon and lime juice with the vinegar. Add the sugar; stir until dissolved. Add the cabbage, cucumber, onion, red pepper and the remaining 1/2 cup each of cilantro and mint and toss well.
- In a shallow bowl, mix the remaining 1/2 cup of panko with the sesame seeds. Pat the mixture onto the salmon burgers.
- In each of 2 large non-stick skillets, heat 2 tablespoons of the oil until shimmering. Add 3 salmon burgers to each skillet and cook over moderately high heat, turning once, until well browned but barely cooked in the center, about 7 minutes.
- Spread the Avocado Aioli on the rolls. Add the salmon burgers, top with the slaw, close the sandwiches and serve.
- MAKE AHEAD: The uncooked salmon burgers and the slaw can be refrigerated overnight.

- NOTES: Sambal is a condiment used in Indonesia, Malaysia, Singapore, the southern Philippines and Sri Lanka, as well as the Netherlands and in Suriname, made from a variety of peppers, although chili peppers are the most common. Sambal is used as a condiment or as a side dish, and is sometimes substituted for fresh chilies; it can be very hot for the uninitiated. It is available at exotic food markets or gourmet departments in supermarkets in numerous countries.

226. Pan Seared Tilapia Or Bass With Chile Lime Butter Recipe

Serving: 6 | Prep: | Cook: 15mins | Ready in:

Ingredients

- For chile lime butter:
- 1/2 stick (1/4 cup) unsalted butter, softened
- 1 tablespoon finely chopped shallot
- 1 teaspoon finely grated fresh lime zest
- 2 teaspoons fresh lime juice
- 1 teaspoon minced fresh Thai or serrano chile (preferably red), including seeds
- 1/2 teaspoon salt
- ****
- For fish:
- 6 (5- to 6-oz) pieces skinless tilapia fillet or farm-raised striped bass fillets with skin
- 1/2 teaspoon salt
- 2 tablespoons vegetable oil

Direction

- Make chile lime butter:
- Stir together butter, shallot, zest, lime juice, chile, and salt in a bowl.
- ****
- Prepare fish:
- If using striped bass, score skin in 3 or 4 places with a thin sharp knife to prevent fish from curling (do not cut through flesh). Pat fish dry and sprinkle with salt. Heat 1 tablespoon oil in a 12-inch nonstick skillet over moderately high heat until just smoking, then sauté 3 pieces of fish, turning over once with a spatula, until golden and just cooked through, 4 to 5 minutes, and transfer to a plate. Sauté remaining fish in remaining tablespoon oil in same manner.
- Serve each piece of fish with a dollop of chile lime butter.
- **NOTE: Chile lime butter can be made 1 day ahead and chilled, covered. Bring to room temperature before using.
- Enjoy.

227. Parmesan Crusted Tilapia Recipe

Serving: 2 | Prep: | Cook: 15mins | Ready in:

Ingredients

- 1 cup of parmesan cheese, grated
- 1/2 cup of Bisquick for the Parmesan mix
- 2 tilapia fillets (5 or 6 oz each)
- Bisquick for dredging
- 1 egg - wisked
- 1 tablespoon of garlic - chopped
- 1 tablespoon of olive oil
- 2 tablespoons of white wine
- 1 tablespoon of capers, drained
- 1/4 cup of chicken stock
- ½ lemon
- salt
- pepper
- 1 tablespoon of butter

Direction

- Mix parmesan cheese with 1/2 cup of bisquick in a shallow pan. In another dish, beat the egg slightly.
- Dredge the Tilapia fillets in plain bisquick. Shake off any surplus flour from the fillets

them dip them in egg then dip them in the Parmesan bisquick mix.

- Heat olive oil in a non-stick frying pan. Place the Parmesan crusted Tilapia fillets in the frying pan and fry them until they are brown on both sides - about 3-4 min. Remove the fillets from the pan and keep them warm.
- Add some more olive oil to the pan and sauté the garlic in the oil.
- Add white wine, capers and chicken stock to the frying pan. Squeeze lemon juice from the lemon over the frying pan and season with salt and pepper and allow the sauce to reduce by half
- Remove the sauce from the heat and add the butter, mix well.
- Place the Parmesan crusted Tilapia fillets on serving dishes and pour sauce over them. Enjoy!

228. Parmesan Puffed Tilapia Recipe

Serving: 4 | Prep: | Cook: 15mins | Ready in:

Ingredients

- 2/3 cup shredded parmesan cheese
- 1/3 cup mayonnaise
- 2 tbsp thinly sliced green onion
- 1/4 tsp hot sauce
- 1 lb tilapia fillets, thawed if frozen
- 1/4 tsp paprika

Direction

- Preheat oven to 375 degrees. Blend Parmesan, mayonnaise, green onion and hot sauce in a small bowl; set aside.
- Pat fish dry with paper towels. Coast a shallow baking dish with non-stick cooking spray; place fillets in baking dish. Spread Parmesan mixture evenly over fillets and sprinkle with paprika.
- Bake 15 to 20 minutes or until fish flakes easily with a fork and topping is puffed and light golden brown.

229. Pastry Wrapped Salmon The One That Got Away With A Side Of Green Beans And Shitake Mushrooms With Kalamata Dressing Recipe

Serving: 4 | Prep: | Cook: 30mins | Ready in:

Ingredients

- Two 8 oz piece of wild caught Sockeye salmon
- 2 cups flour
- 1 tsp. salt
- 3/4 c. butter
- ¼cup plus 3 tablespoons ice water
- Egg Wash:
- One egg slightly beaten and two tablespoons of water.
- For the green beans:
- 1/3 cup pitted kalamata olives
- 1/4 cup lightly packed fresh parsley leaves, plus 1 Tbs. roughly chopped
- 1/4 cup mayonnaise
- 3 medium cloves garlic, peeled
- kosher salt and freshly ground black pepper
- 4 oz of shitake mushrooms sliced into ¼-inch slices
- 1-tablespoon olive oil
- sea salt to taste
- ¼-teaspoon fresh ground black pepper.
- 2 lb. green beans trimmed

Direction

- Make the dough ahead and chill before rolling.
- Roll the dough as if making a piecrust. Roll around the clock. Start with the rolling pin in the center of your dough disk. Roll toward 12 o'clock, easing up on the pressure as you near the edge (this keeps the edge from getting too

thin). Pick up the pin and return it to center. Roll toward 6 o'clock, as shown at right. Repeat this motion toward 3 and then 9 o'clock, always easing up the pressure near the edges and then picking up the pin rather than rolling it back to center. Continue to roll around the clock, aiming for different "times" (like 1, 7, 4, and 10) on each round

- Turn the dough and check often for sticking. After each round of the clock, run a bench knife underneath the dough (below left), to make sure it is not sticking, and reflour the surface if necessary. When you do this, give the dough a quarter turn – most people inevitably use uneven pressure when rolling in one direction versus another, so the occasional turn helps average it out for a more even thickness. Continue to turn and roll until the dough is the right width and thickness. For this, I rolled it out to about 1/8 inch "on the plus side"
- Trim off edges so you have a rectangle and use the scraps for your decorations.
- Place salmon onto dough with two inches of boarder and fold over dough tuck the dough with your hand around the salmon.
- Cut a tail shape and fin outline at the top and shape of a fish head with a sharp knife.
- Seal the edges by hand all around "lightly" pressing the edge with your fingers
- With a fork, seal the tail and top fin.
- Cut out the fins and make fork mark then attach to the body of the fish using a little water on the back of the fin.
- Make a small eye from the dough, wet it, and attach it to the dough.
- Cut a vent hole in the shape of a gill in the dough and lift slightly with the knife.
- Place on parchment paper lined cookie sheet and brush on egg wash.
- Bake for twenty minutes until lightly browned.
- In the meantime, make the green beans.
- Olive mixture:
- Put the olives, parsley leaves, mayonnaise, garlic, a pinch of sea salt and 1/4 tsp. pepper in a food processor and pulse into a coarse paste set aside the dressing.
- Green beans:
- Bring a large pot of well-salted water to a boil.
- Working in 3 batches, boil the green beans until tender, about 5 minutes per batch.
- Drain each batch well and keep warm in a large bowl covered with foil.
- In a small fry pan sauté the shitake mushrooms in one tablespoons of olive oil until tender add a pinch of salt and sauté a few minutes more add to the green beans and toss to combine.
- Dab the olive mixture over the green beans and toss well to combine.
- Season to taste with salt and pepper. Transfer to a platter, sprinkle with the chopped parsley, and serve.
- Make Ahead Tips
- The kalamata olive dressing can be made 1 day ahead and refrigerated until ready to use.
- Plate your pastry wrapped salmon and serve immediately.
- Serve with the green beans in a separate dish.

230. Pecan Crusted Salmon Recipe

Serving: 8 | Prep: | Cook: 15mins | Ready in:

Ingredients

- salmon
- 8 portions of salmon fillets cut in 4-5 oz. portions
- 2 cups pecans
- 1 Tbs. garlic
- 1/2 tsp. salt
- 1/4 tsp. cayenne
- 1/2 cup extra virgin olive oil
- mango SALSA RECIPE
- 2 ripe mangos, skinned and cubed
- 1/2 cup red onions, small diced
- 1 tsp. orange zest

- 1 finely diced poblano pepper
- 1 diced red bell pepper
- shot of orange juice
- shot of red wine vinegar
- 1 bunch chopped cilantro
- TO SERVE
- 1 1/2 pounds baby greens
- olive oil
- balsamic vinegar

Direction

- SALMON
- Grind pecans in to a coarse meal.
- Add all ingredients together.
- Dip salmon fillets in olive oil and roll in pecan crumb mixture.
- Heat a large fry pan and lightly sauté the salmon on one side.
- Turn onto a sheet pan and roast fish in a 450 degree F oven for 4-5 minutes or until done to taste.
- Flip the fish about halfway through baking.
- Check that there's still wine in the dish, as this keeps it from drying out
- Fish is done when skin is loose to the touch and meat in the thickest part has turned from translucent to pink or white, and is slightly flaky.
- MANGO SALSA
- Mix all ingredients together and let sit for 2 hours.
- TO SERVE
- Toss greens in 1 teaspoon each of olive oil and balsamic vinegar.
- Add pinch of salt.
- Place greens on each plate.
- Top with salmon, then top with salsa and serve.
- Serve with rice.

231. Pecan Crusted Catfish Recipe

Serving: 4 | Prep: | Cook: 25mins | Ready in:

Ingredients

- 1/2 cup buttermilk
- 1/4 tps. hot sauce
- 1/2 tps. dried oregano
- 1/2 tps. chili powder
- 1/4 tps. garlic powder
- 2 cups cornflakes
- 1/2 cup pecan pieces
- 1 pound catfish fillets, about 1 inch thick, cut into 4 portions

Direction

- Preheat oven to 375F. Line a baking sheet with foil.
- Blend buttermilk, hot sauce, oregano, chili powder and garlic powder in a shallow dish. Pulse cornflakes in a food processor until coarse crumbs form. Transfer to a large plate. Pulse pecans in the food processor until coarsely chopped; mix the pecans with the cornflake crumbs.
- Dip each catfish fillet in the buttermilk mixture, then dredge in the cornflake mixture, coating both sides. Transfer to the prepared baking sheet.
- Bake the catfish for 25 minutes, or until it flakes easily with a fork.

232. Peppered Haddock With Garlic Whipped Potatoes And Parsley Sauce Recipe

Serving: 12 | Prep: | Cook: 14mins | Ready in:

Ingredients

- 12 oz olive oil
- 1 oz lemon juice

- 1/2 cup Chopped parsley
- 1/2 tsp salt
- 3 1/2 lb haddock fillets cut into 5-oz portions
- 2 tbsp Crushed black peppercorns
- 2 1/2 oz garlic Whipped potatoes

Direction

- Prepare the sauce:
- Combine 10 oz. oil, lemon juice, chopped parsley, and salt in a blender.
- Process until the parsley is puréed.
- Coat the fish fillets evenly with a light sprinkling of crushed peppercorns.
- Season with salt.
- Heat 2 oz. olive oil in as many sauté pans as necessary to hold the fish in a single layer.
- Place the fish in the pans, presentation side down, and sauté over moderate heat until lightly browned and about half cooked.
- Turn over and finish the cooking.
- Place a 3-oz portion of potatoes in the center of each plate.
- Top with the fish fillet.
- Drizzle about 1 oz. sauce in a circle around the fish.
- ========================
- Variations:
- Other firm-fleshed white fish, such as cod, sea bass, striped bass, red snapper, or grouper, may be substituted.

233. Peppered Tuna Steaks With Korean Style Salad Recipe

Serving: 4 | Prep: | Cook: 20mins | Ready in:

Ingredients

- 1/2 cup shredded napa cabbage
- 1/4 cup fresh bean sprouts
- 1 cucumber peeled seeded and thinly sliced
- 1/4 cup soy sauce
- 1/4 cup rice vinegar
- 1 tablespoon minced ginger
- 1 tablespoon minced garlic
- 1 fresh chili pepper of your choice minced
- 2 tablespoons granulated sugar
- 2 tablespoons roughly chopped fresh basil
- salt and pepper to taste
- Tuna:
- 4 fresh tuna steaks
- 1/4 cup coarsely ground peppercorns
- 1/2 teaspoon kosher salt

Direction

- In medium bowl, combine cabbage, bean sprouts and cucumber.
- Combine soy sauce, vinegar, ginger, garlic, chili pepper, sugar, basil, salt and pepper.
- Whisk together well then add just enough to cabbage mixture to moisten ingredients.
- Toss well then cover and refrigerate.
- Preheat broiler to high then rub tuna all over with ground peppercorns and sprinkle with salt.
- Place on a lightly greased broiler pan and broil until done to your liking about 6 minutes per side.
- Distribute salad among 4 plates then top each with a tuna steak and serve at once.

234. Pescespada Stemperata Swordfish Stemperata Recipe

Serving: 4 | Prep: | Cook: 10mins | Ready in:

Ingredients

- 1/4 cup extra virgin olive oil
- Four 6 to 8-ounce swordfish steaks (3/4 inch thickness)
- All purpose flour
- 1 onion, finely chopped
- 1 and 1/3 cups pitted Spanish green olives, quartered lengthwise

- 1/2 cup golden raisins
- 1/4 cup drained capers
- 1/4 cup white wine vinegar
- 1/4 cup minced fresh mint

Direction

- Heat olive oil in heavy large skillet over high heat.
- Season fish with salt and pepper. Coat fish in flour and add to skillet. Cook until brown, about 2 minutes per side. Transfer fish to plate.
- Add onion to same skillet, reduce heat to medium and cook until golden, about 4 minutes.
- Add olives, raisins and capers. Reduce heat to low; cook 2 minutes, stirring frequently.
- Return fish to skillet.
- Spoon sautéed ingredients over. Add vinegar and half of mint; cook until fish is cooked through, about 2 minutes.
- Season with salt and pepper.
- Transfer fish to plates, spooning sautéed ingredients over. Sprinkle with remaining mint.

235. Pineapple Teriyaki Salmon Recipe

Serving: 4 | Prep: | Cook: 20mins |Ready in:

Ingredients

- 2 tablespoons brown sugar
- 2 tablespoons low-sodium soy sauce
- 1 teaspoon finely grated orange zest
- 1 (6-ounce) can pineapple juice
- 1/2 teaspoon salt, divided
- 2 teaspoons canola oil
- 4 (6-ounce) salmon fillets (about 1 inch thick)
- 1/4 teaspoon freshly ground black pepper
- Grated orange rind (optional)

Direction

- Combine first 4 ingredients and 1/4 teaspoon salt in a small saucepan over high heat, and bring to a boil. Reduce heat, and simmer until reduced to 1/4 cup (about 15 minutes). Set aside.
- Preheat oven to 400 degrees F.
- Heat oil in a large non-stick skillet over medium-high heat. Sprinkle both sides of salmon with remaining 1/4 teaspoon salt and black pepper. Add fish to pan; cook 3 minutes. Turn fish over and place in oven; bake at 400 degrees F for 3 minutes. Remove from oven; brush 1 tablespoon sauce over each fillet. Return to oven, and cook 1 minute or until fish flakes easily when tested with a fork or until desired degree of doneness. Sprinkle with orange rind, if desired.

236. Pistachio Crusted Halibut With Spicy Yogurt Recipe

Serving: 4 | Prep: | Cook: 10mins |Ready in:

Ingredients

- For halibut
- 4 (1 1/4-inch-thick) pieces skinless halibut fillet (about 6 oz each)
- 1 cup whole milk
- 1/3 cup shelled pistachios (preferably Turkish), finely chopped
- 3 tablespoons cornmeal
- 3/4 teaspoon salt
- 1/4 teaspoon black pepper
- 1/4 cup extra-virgin olive oil
- For Spicy yogurt
- 1 cup thick Turkish or Greek yogurt (8 oz)
- 1/2 cucumber, peeled, seeded, and finely diced (3/4 cup)
- 2 tablespoons chopped fresh dill
- 1 tablespoon finely chopped onion
- 1 tablespoon fresh lemon juice
- 2 teaspoons dried maras pepper
- 1/2 teaspoon salt, or to taste

Direction

- Put fish in a shallow baking dish, pour milk over it, and chill, covered, turning over once, 30 minutes. 3Meanwhile, stir together pistachios and cornmeal in a shallow bowl.
- Remove fish from milk, letting excess drip off. Transfer to a plate and sprinkle all over with salt and pepper, then dredge lightly in cornmeal-pistachio mixture. Transfer to a clean plate as coated.
- Heat oil in a 12-inch heavy skillet over moderately high heat until hot but not smoking, then sauté fish, turning over once, until golden and just cooked through, 6 to 8 minutes total.
- While fish cooks, stir together all ingredients for spicy yogurt.
- Serve fish with spicy yogurt on the side.
- Cooks' note: If you can't find Turkish or Greek yogurt, use regular plain whole-milk yogurt drained in a sieve or colander lined with a double thickness of paper towels, chilled, 1 hour.

237. Planked Salmon With Cucumber Dill Sauce Recipe

Serving: 4 | Prep: | Cook: 20mins | Ready in:

Ingredients

- 1 /12 lbs salmon filets, skin on
- 2 Tbl olive oil
- 2 Tbl brown sugar
- 2 garlic cloves, minced
- 2 tsp dried dill, divided
- 1 medium cucumber, peeled, seede and thinly sliced
- 2 Tbl plain yougurt or sour cream
- 1 tsp white wine vinegar

Direction

- Submerge cedar plank in cold water at least an hour or overnight.
- Brush skin side of fillets and place in a large.
- In a small bowl, combine brown sugar, garlic and 1 tsp of the dill.
- Spread mixture over salmon, pressing to coat.
- Cover and refrigerate at least one hour.
- Preheat grill to medium low.
- Place plank on grill and heat until they begin to smoke, about 5 minutes.
- Season salmon with salt and pepper to taste and place skin side down on plank.
- Grill covered about 20 minutes or until fish slakes easily with a fork.
- Meanwhile, for sauce, in a small bowl combine remaining dill, cucumber, yogurt or sour cream, vinegar and salt and pepper to taste; stir, chill, serve with salmon.

238. Poached Curry Halibut Recipe

Serving: 4 | Prep: | Cook: 10mins | Ready in:

Ingredients

- 1 pound halibut, sea bass or other firm thick white fish, cut into 4 ounce portions (skin and bones removed please)
- 1 1/2 cups fumet, (fish stock) or, clam juice
- 1/2 cup heavy cream
- 2 tablespoons fine curry powder (I found one at a little farmer's market called lemon curry powder, that was soooo good, but I've made this with others and they turn out good too), or to taste
- 1 teaspoon fresh lemon juice
- 1 teaspoon cornstarch mixed with 1 teaspoon water, (to thicken the sauce, optional, but I like a nice thick sauce)
- Optional toppers, optional yes, but good none the less
- toasted coconut
- chopped peanuts or cashews

- thinly sliced green onion tops
- golden raisins

Direction

- Heat oven to 350 degrees F.
- Place the fish stock, cream and curry into an ovenproof sauté pan and bring to a boil. Reduce heat to a simmer. Season the fish with salt and pepper (white pepper works well here) and place in the curry mixture, turning to cover the fish with sauce. Cover the pan and pop it into the oven. Cook for 5 - 7 minutes (depending on thickness of fish) or until JUST cooked through. Do NOT overcook the fish.
- Remove fish, cover lightly with foil. Bring the sauce to a boil over a medium heat and either allow to reduce slightly or add your cornstarch slush. Stir until thickened. Stir in lemon juice.
- Place the fish on top of plain boiled or steamed white rice. Spoon the sauce over and sprinkle with condiments of choice.
- Per Serving (without rice or condiments) 236 Calories; 12g Fat (6g Sat, 4g Mono, 1g Poly); 25g Protein; 2g Carbohydrate; trace Dietary Fiber; 68mg Cholesterol; 161mg Sodium.

239. Poached Fingers Of Salmon And Turbot With Saffron And Julienne Of Vegetables Recipe

Serving: 10 | Prep: | Cook: 30mins | Ready in:

Ingredients

- 8 oz leeks
- 8 oz carrots
- 8 oz celery or celery root
- 8 oz onion sliced thin
- 2 1/2 qt water, cold
- to taste --- salt pepper
- 2 1/4 lb Turbot fillets
- 2 1/4 lb salmon fillets
- pinch --- saffron threads
- 1 oz Chopped chives

Direction

- Cut the leeks, carrots, and celery or celery root into julienne and keep the trimmings.
- Place the trimmings into a deep pan with the onion and cover with the water.
- Bring slowly to a boil and skim to remove any impurities.
- Simmer for 30 minutes, then strain into a shallow poaching pan and keep barely simmering to reduce to 1 1/2 of its original volume.
- Season to preference.
- Skin the fillets.
- Cut the fish into pieces, 1 × 4 in. and add to the cooking liquid with the vegetable strips and saffron.
- Simmer for 5 minutes.
- Check the seasoning.
- Serve in broad soup plates with the cooking liquid.
- Sprinkle with chopped chives.

240. Poached Salmon With Cucumber Lemon Sauce Recipe

Serving: 4 | Prep: | Cook: 10mins | Ready in:

Ingredients

- 1 quart water
- ½ cup white wine
- 1 small onion, quartered and sliced lengthwise
- 1 teaspoon salt
- 10 peppercorns
- 4 (6-oz) salmon steaks
- cucumber-Lemon Sauce:
- 1 large cucumber, peeled and seeded
- salt
- ¼ cup mayonnaise

- ¼ cup sour cream
- 1 teaspoon grated lemon peel
- 1 tablespoon lemon juice
- 1 teaspoon minced onion

Direction

- Combine water, wine, onion, salt and peppercorns in large skillet.
- Bring to boil.
- Add salmon steaks and return to boil.
- Reduce heat and simmer, covered, until salmon flakes easily when tested with fork, about 10 minutes.
- Remove steaks and drain.
- Serve with Cucumber-Lemon sauce.
- ****
- Cucumber-lemon Sauce:
- Shred cucumber and sprinkle lightly with salt.
- Let stand 30 minutes.
- Drain, squeezing to remove excess liquid.
- Place cucumber in bowl.
- Add mayonnaise, sour cream, lemon peel, lemon juice and onion and stir to blend.
- Taste and add more salt if needed.
- Makes 1 cup.

241. Poached Salmon With Melon Salsa Recipe

Serving: 6 | Prep: | Cook: 15mins | Ready in:

Ingredients

- 2 green onions, thinly sliced, including green portions
- 1 1/2 tsp. fresh mint, chopped
- 1 tsp. fresh ginger, grated
- 3 Tbsp. grated lime zest
- 1 1/2 lbs. salmon fillets, skinned and cut into 6 pieces
- melon salsa......
- 1 honeydew melon, about 3 lbs., peeled, seeded and cut into 1/2-inch cubes
- 1 yellow bell pepper, seeded, stemmed and cut into 1/2-inch squares
- 1/4 cup lime juice
- 1/2 red onion, chopped
- 1 jalapeno chili, minced
- 2 Tbsp. fresh mint, chopped

Direction

- Preheat oven at 450 F.
- In a small bowl, toss together onion, mint, ginger and lime zest.
- Place 6 pieces of aluminum foil, each 10 inches square, on a work surface. Place a piece of salmon in the center of each square.
- Top each with an equal amount of onion mixture.
- Fold in the edges of foil and crimp to seal.
- Place the packets in a single layer on a baking sheet and bake until opaque throughout, 12 to 15 minutes.
- Meanwhile, to make salsa, in a medium bowl, toss together the melon, pepper, lime juice, onion, jalapeno and mint.
- To serve, transfer the contents of each packet onto an individual plate.
- Top each with an equal amount of the salsa.

242. Prosciutto Frizzled Fish Recipe

Serving: 4 | Prep: | Cook: 25mins | Ready in:

Ingredients

- For bread Crumbs:
- 2 oz. prosciutto,diced (1/2 c)
- 2 Tbs extra virgin olive oil
- 1 c fresh bread crumbs
- 1 Tbs chopped fresh parsley
- 1 tsp minced lemon zest
- salt and red pepper flakes to taste
- For the Fish:
- 4 white fish fillets,such as halibut,cod,tilapia seasoned with salt and pepper(4-6 oz ea.)

- 2 Tbs extra virgin olive oil
- 12 thin lemon slices
- Prepared bread crumbs

Direction

- Preheat oven to 400 degrees. Sauté prosciutto for the bread crumbs in 2 tbsp oil in sauté pan over med-high heat until crisp, 5 mins. Drain on paper-towel-lined plate.
- Toast crumbs in the prosciutto drippings in same pan over med-high heat till browned, 2 mins. Combine with parsley, zest, prosciutto, salt and pepper flakes; set aside.
- Sear fish in 2 tbsp oil in ovenproof skillet over med-high heat. Carefully flip fillets over and transfer pan to the oven. Roast fish until fillets flake easily with fork, 5-6 mins.
- To serve, mound some garlicky spinach on each plate and top with lemon slices and a fillet. Garnish with bread crumbs.
- Garlicky spinach;
- 2 tbsp chopped garlic
- 1 tsp red pepper flakes
- 1 tbsp extra virgin olive oil
- 1 bag fresh spinach (9oz0
- Salt to taste
- Sauté garlic and red pepper flakes in oil in large sauté pan over med-high heat until fragrant, 30 secs to 1 min. Add the spinach and toss with tongs to wilt, 2 mins. Season with salt.

243. Real English Fish And Chips With Beer Batter Recipe

Serving: 4 | Prep: | Cook: 1hours | Ready in:

Ingredients

- • 4 cod fish fillets.
- • ¾ cup plain flour.
- • 1 tsp. bicarbonate of soda (baking soda).
- • 8 fluid ounce (235 ml) beer.
- • Juice of ½ lemon.
- • Salt & pepper, to taste.
- • Extra flour
- • 3 lb. (1.5 kg.) potatoes, peeled & sliced into chips (French fries).
- • Good quality cooking oil, to make 4 inches (25 cm) in your pot or wok.
- • Malt vinegar. And lemon wedges for serving.

Direction

- Heat oil in a pot, wok or deep fat fryer to 375 F (190°C.).
- Peel the potatoes and cut into chips. Rinse and dry thoroughly.
- Fry chips for about 3 minutes until soft but NOT colored.
- Drain and shake well and set to one side.
- Put some flour onto a plate. Dredge the Cod fillets in the flour thoroughly - this is VERY important, it stops the batter sliding off when the fish is fried! Leave the fish fillets in the flour whilst you make the batter.
- Some people say you should make the batter at least one hour before, I can't tell any difference. Make it before if it is convenient or now!
- Put flour, bicarbonate of soda, salt and pepper into a large roomy bowl.
- Add the beer gradually, until you have a thick, coating type batter. Drink any beer that's left!
- Whisk batter thoroughly until it is smooth and there are no lumps.
- Add the lemon juice or a splash of malt vinegar if desired. Mix thoroughly again.
- Have your plates, newspaper or whatever ready for serving!
- Adjust the cooking oil temp to 325 F. (160°C.).
- Take one fillet of fish at a time and holding it by the tail or thin end (!) swirl it around the batter until well coated, plunge into hot oil immediately.
- As soon as it has crisped up and sets, add your other fillets one at a time, taking out the first ones as they cook, about 6 to 10 minutes, depending on the thickness. Turn if necessary.
- Place onto a tray and keep warm in the oven.

- Turn up the heat setting to 190°C again and cook your chips until golden and crisp.
- Serve on plates or newspaper with salt, lemon wedges & vinegar!
- If you just have to have mayo or Tartar sauce, go for it. I don't use it unless I'm forced to eat, dry a buggery, tuna fish and chips. With Cod you just need lemon juice and Malt vinegar.

244. Red Lobsters Salmon With Lobster Mashed Potatoes Recipe

Serving: 4 | Prep: | Cook: 45mins | Ready in:

Ingredients

- Ingredients:
- * 4 eight-to-ten ounce pieces of fresh salmon fillets, skinless
- * ½ cup canola oil
- * McCormick's season All
- * 4 heaping portions of your favorite mashed potato recipe
- * Fresh vegetables of your choice (asparagus is a nice touch)
- * 2 tbsp. chopped fresh parsley
- * 2 tbsp. chopped green onions
- * 4 lemon wedges
- lobster Sauce
- * 1 live Maine lobster, 1 ¼ pound
- * 1 quart heavy whipping cream
- * 1 medium onion, diced
- * 2 stalks celery, diced
- * 2 carrots, peeled and diced
- * 1 bay leaf
- * 1 tsp. black peppercorns, whole
- * ¼ cup flour, all purpose
- * ½ cup butter, salted
- * 2 tbsps. tomato paste
- * ½ cup cream sherry
- * 1 tsp. fresh thyme leaves, stem removed
- * salt and fresh-ground black pepper

Direction

- Lobster Sauce
- Prepare lobster by cutting in half lengthwise through the head and body first. Remove tail halves, and claw and knuckle sections. These are the sections with the meat for the sauce. Cut the body into two-inch pieces.
- In a two-quart stock pot heat the butter over medium heat. Add all diced vegetables, lobster, peppercorns, bay leaf, and thyme. Cook on medium to medium-high heat, stirring continually for ten minutes or until the lobster shells start to turn red. Remove just the lobster pieces that contain meat and let cool for ten minutes.
- Stir in flour and cook on medium heat, stirring continually for another 5 minutes.
- Deglaze pan with sherry, then add cream.
- Remove lobster meat from the shell, and set aside. Place leftover shells back into the lobster cream. Let reduce on low heat to desired consistency. (We suggest thick enough to coat the back of a spoon.)
- Cut lobster meat into half-inch chunks.
- Strain lobster sauce into a smaller pot and discard shell/vegetable mixture.
- Stir in lobster meat and season sauce to taste with salt and pepper just before serving.
- Grilled Salmon
- Lightly brush both sides of fillets with olive oil and season with McCormick's Season All.
- Pre-heat grill on medium-high heat and place salmon on, skin-side up. Grill for 4-5 minutes until well-marked.
- Turn fish over and continue grilling another 5-6 minutes or until your fresh fish preference is reached.

245. Red Snapper Mediterranean Style Recipe

Serving: 4 | Prep: | Cook: 20mins | Ready in:

Ingredients

- 4 x 6oz Skin on Fillets Of American Red or Pacific Snapper
- 12 pieces Baby fennel
- 2 cups chicken stock
- 1 # spinach, cleaned
- 8 Vine Ripe tomatoes, peeled, seeded and diced 2 lemons
- 1/8 cup
- sugar
- 1/4 cup olive oil
- Cracked black peppercorns
- sea salt
- Chopped fresh herbs (parsley, chervil, tarragon and basil)

Direction

- Method
- Braise the baby fennel in the chicken stock until tender. Keep fennel in the broth and cool.
- Toss diced tomatoes with sea salt and pepper to taste.
- Peel the lemon zest and blanch in cold water making sure the peel is only the yellow and not the white pith.
- Boil the water with sugar and make a heavy syrup. Cook lemon peel in the syrup until the peel is candied and translucent. Set aside to cool and then finely julienne the peel. Reserve the syrup.
- Season the red snapper fillets. Heat a heavy sauté pan and sear the fish in half the amount of olive oil. Cook flesh-side first and give the fish a good color. Cook fish in the skin and crisp the skin. Cook fish until tender, about 8 minutes.
- Wash spinach thoroughly. Place spinach leaves on a plate. Place fish on top of spinach. Sauté the tomatoes in the remaining olive oil. Add the fennel bulbs which have now been split in half lengthwise. Add two spoons of chopped fresh herbs and the lemon zest. Taste for seasonings.
- Finish dish with a tablespoon of the lemon syrup and a quarter cup of the fennel braising broth.
- Heat up plates in the oven. Arrange six pieces of fennel on each plate. Spoon tomato relish on top of the fish and lightly drizzle the broth over the top. Garnish with sprigs of tarragon and chervil.

246. Red Snapper Veracruz Recipe

Serving: 4 | Prep: | Cook: 30mins | Ready in:

Ingredients

- 4 red snapper filets
- 1/2 tsp adobo seasoning
- 2 limes (juice of)
- 2 tbls olive oil
- 1 med onion, sliced into rings
- 2 cloves garlic minced
- 3 jalapeno peppers,seeded cut into strips
- 1 large tomato,seeded cut into strips
- 3tbls tomato paste
- 1/8 tsp dried oregano
- 1/2 cup white wine
- 1 cup clam broth (juice)
- 2 tbls spanish capers
- 1/2 cup Spanish olives with pimientos
- 4 cups cooked rice

Direction

- Season fish with adobo and lime juice.Set aside. In a skillet, heat oil on medium heat. Stir in onion until translucent. Stir in garlic and jalapenos cook for 2 min. Stir in tomatoes and tomato paste, wine, broth bring to boil. Stir in capers and olives. Add fish filets and cover with sauce. Cook until fish will flake with fork about 8 min. Serve with rice.

247. Red Snapper Veracruz Style Huachinango A La Veracruzana Recipe

Serving: 6 | Prep: | Cook: 35mins | Ready in:

Ingredients

- For Sauce:
- 1 28-ounce can diced tomatoes in juice, well drained, juices reserved
- 1/4 cup extra-virgin olive oil
- 1/4 cup finely chopped white onion
- 3 large garlic cloves, chopped
- 3 small bay leaves
- 2 tablespoons chopped fresh parsley
- 1 teaspoon dried Mexican oregano
- 1/4 cup chopped pitted green olives
- 2 tablespoons raisins
- 2 tablespoons drained capers
- ~~~~
- 6 4- to 5-ounce red snapper fillets
- 3 pickled jalapeño chiles, halved lengthwise

Direction

- Make Sauce:
- Place drained tomatoes in medium bowl. Using potato masher, crush tomatoes to coarse puree. Drain again, reserving juices.
- Heat oil in heavy large skillet over medium-high heat.
- Add onion and stir 30 seconds. Add garlic and stir 30 seconds.
- Add tomato puree and cook 1 minute. Add bay leaves, parsley, oregano, and 1/4 cup reserved tomato juices. Simmer until sauce thickens, about 3 minutes.
- Add olives, raisins, capers, and all remaining reserved tomato juices. Simmer until sauce thickens again, stirring occasionally, about 8 minutes.
- Season sauce to taste with salt and pepper. (Can be made 1 day ahead. Cover and refrigerate.)
- ~~~~
- Cook Fish:
- Preheat oven to 425°F.
- Spread 3 tablespoons sauce in bottom of 15x10x2-inch glass baking dish.
- Arrange fish atop sauce. Sprinkle fish lightly with salt and pepper.
- Spoon remaining sauce over.
- Bake uncovered until fish is just opaque in center, about 18 minutes.
- Using long spatula, transfer fish with sauce to plates. Garnish with pickled jalapeño halves.

248. Red Snapper With Garlic And Lime Recipe

Serving: 0 | Prep: | Cook: 12mins | Ready in:

Ingredients

- 2-6 (8oz) snapper fillets
- 1/2 cup chopped cilantro
- 1.5 tablespoons minced garlic
- 1.5 tablespoons finely grated fresh lime zest
- 6 tablespoons extra-virgin olive oil
- 3/4 teaspoon black pepper
- 1 teaspoon salt

Direction

- Preheat your broiler and prepare a shallow baking pan with a small amount of oil.
- Pat the fish dry and place with skin side up into the pan. Take 3 teaspoons of olive oil and brush *both* sides of the fish. Sprinkle a little salt and pepper on top.
- Place the fish *6 inches* away from the heat source. Broil for about 10 minutes.
- While that is cooking, toss up cilantro, garlic and zest in a bowl.
- Remove fish and sprinkle with the cilantro-garlic-zest mixture. You can optionally drizzle a little olive oil on top at the end.

249. Red Snapper With Orange Plum Sauce Recipe

Serving: 4 | Prep: | Cook: 20mins | Ready in:

Ingredients

- 4 red snapper fillets
- 2 Tbsp soy sauce
- 1/2 cup all-purpose flour
- 1/4 tsp salt
- 1/8 tsp black pepper
- 2 to 3 Tbsp plus 1 tsp peanut oil
- 1/2 cup orange juice
- 1 tsp cornstarch
- 2 Tbsp minced garlic
- 1 jalapeno pepper, seeded & minced
- 1/2 cup plum sauce
- 2 Tbsp rice wine
- 1 Tbsp chili garlic sauce
- 1 Tbsp minced green onion, green part only (optional)

Direction

- Combine snapper fillets and soy sauce in Ziploc; turn to coat all sides. Let stand 30 minutes
- Combine flour, salt & pepper on shallow plate. Remove fish from soy sauce; coat with flour mixture
- Heat 2 Tbsp oil in large nonstick skillet. Place fish and cook over medium-high heat 4 to 5 minutes per side.
- Remove fish from skillet and keep warm.
- While fish is cooking, stir orange juice into cornstarch in small bowl; mix well.
- Heat 1 tsp oil in small saucepan over medium-high heat. Add garlic & jalapeno pepper; cook and stir 1 to 2 minutes.
- Add cornstarch mixture, plum sauce, rice wine and chili garlic sauce; cook and stir a couple minutes or until slightly thickened.
- Arrange fish on plates and top with sauce; garnish with green onion.

250. Riviera Flounder Recipe

Serving: 4 | Prep: | Cook: 15mins | Ready in:

Ingredients

- 8 small to medium flounder fillets (2 each)
- 1- 2 tbsp of mild veggie oil
- 1/2 to 3/4 cup of slivered fennel (bulb part on mandolin)
- 1 can of diced tomatoes, drained
- 1/3 cup or so of chopped green olives stuffed with pimentos
- 1/3 cup of white vermouth
- 1 onion sliced thinly lengthwise-mimic the fennel shape
- 1 garlic clove minced
- 5 strips of orange zest, julienned
- juice of one half of orange
- pinch or two of red pepper flakes, more if desired
- pinch of dried parsley flakes
- large pinch of dried tarragon leaves
- 1 tbsp of capers
- 1 tbsp of butter

Direction

- Heat oil in large flat skillet.
- Quickly sauté salt and peppered fish fillets. About 3 minutes per side. Reserve, tent with foil to keep warm.
- In the pan drippings quickly cook the fennel, onion and garlic with a touch of oil if it seems to dry, until just tender.
- Add vermouth, orange juice and reduce until there is only a tbsp of so of liquid.
- Add seasonings, olives, capers and tomatoes, heat thoroughly about five minutes to meld the flavors.
- Turn off heat, stir in butter to create sauce.
- Pour hot sauce over fish and serve.
- A dish of couscous is a delightful side, along with shredded zucchini in sour cream with nutmeg.

251. Roasted Red Snapper With Lemon Parsley Crumbs Recipe

Serving: 4 | Prep: | Cook: 12mins | Ready in:

Ingredients

- 1 cup panko
- 3 tbsp melted butter
- 3 tbsp chopped parsley
- 2 tsp lemon zest, plus rest of lemon
- salt and pepper
- 1 large red snapper fillet (enough to fed four)

Direction

- Preheat oven to 425, with the rack in the middle.
- In a bowl, combine panko, butter, parsley, lemon zest, salt and pepper.
- Stir to combine.
- Oil a rimmed baking sheet (or use parchment paper).
- Season fish with salt and pepper.
- Place panko topping all over the top of fish and bake for 10-12 minutes.
- Throw under the broiler for about 30 seconds to really crisp up the top.
- Squeeze lemon juice over the top.

252. Roasted Salmon James Bond Recipe

Serving: 6 | Prep: | Cook: 30mins | Ready in:

Ingredients

- The Fish:
- 1 large salmon filet (1 1/-2 lbs)
- The Martini:
- 1 t. dill weed
- juice of ½ lemon
- 1/3 cup vodka
- ¼ cup dry vermouth
- 4 T. melted butter (or more as required)
- 2 t. creamed horseradish
- 1 t. crushed garlic
- 1 t. Tabasco sauce

Direction

- 1 hour before cooking, take salmon from refrigerator. Rinse and pat dry. Remove any pin bones with a tweezers. Put the salmon on a double layer of large aluminum foil sheets. Close it on three sides. Add the "martini". Close the foil tightly. Let stand for 1 hour.
- Prepare a wood fire for indirect cooking.
- Cook the salmon for 30 minutes with foil closed. Carefully open the top. Let the salmon cook for 10-15 minutes longer until sauce reduces. Serve the salmon with the thickened sauce. If the sauce has become too thick, melt an additional tablespoon of butter over salmon.

253. Romanos Macaroni Grill Grilled Salmon With Spinach Orzo Recipe

Serving: 4 | Prep: | Cook: 10mins | Ready in:

Ingredients

- 4 Bias Cut salmon Filets (2 lbs total)
- 1oz canola oil
- 1oz soy sauce
- 8oz Teriyaki glaze (posted below)
- 16oz garlic olive oil sauce
- 4oz Diced red bell peppers
- 24oz orzo pasta, precooked
- 8oz spinach, julienned
- TERIYAKI GLAZE:
- 2 cups soy sauce
- ¾ cups Italian dressing
- 4 cups honey

- ¾ cups lemon juice
- 2 TBSP red pepper, crushed
- 1/8 cup cayenne pepper

Direction

- Dip salmon in soy sauce then the oil.
- Place the salmon on hot grill silver side up.
- Grill salmon evenly until done, approximately 6-7 minutes or until the internal temperature reaches 145 F.
- Slowly ladle the teriyaki glaze over the salmon while still on the grill.
- In a hot sauté pan, add olive oil garlic mix, red bell peppers and orzo.
- At home, an ounce or two of chicken stock will help the orzo during this step.
- Sauté for approximately one minute until orzo is almost dry, stirring to prevent sticking.
- Remove pan from heat and add spinach.
- Toss for approximately three seconds until spinach is incorporated but is not wilted.
- Place spinach and orzo on a plate, then add salmon and additional honey teriyaki glaze if needed.
- TERIYAKI GLAZE
- Mix all ingredients together by hand whisk. Sauce will remain for 48 hours so it needs to be prepared fresh or the day before.

254. SALMON PATTIES Recipe

Serving: 16 | Prep: | Cook: 10mins | Ready in:

Ingredients

- 1 can pink salmon,drained
- 2 eggs
- 1/2 C. chopped onion
- 1/4 to 1/2 C flour
- 2 Tbs. corn meal
- 1/2 tsp. salt

Direction

- Put all ingredients into large mixing bowl except flour.
- Use potato masher to mix to ensure it is mixed well and broken up good.
- While doing this add a little flour at a time until mixture has a good consistency to hold together good.
- Drop into skillet by tablespoon full and pat out with back of spoon.
- Cook over medium heat with plenty of oil until brown on bottom then flip and cook on other side until it is brown.
- Drain on paper towels.

255. Sake Steamed Sea Bass With Ginger And Green Onions Recipe

Serving: 4 | Prep: | Cook: 15mins | Ready in:

Ingredients

- 1 cup uncooked medium-grain rice
- 3/4 cup sake
- 3/4 cup bottled clam juice
- 1 tablespoon minced peeled ginger
- 4 5-ounce sea bass fillets
- 2 large green onions, chopped
- 4 teaspoons soy sauce
- 1 teaspoon oriental sesame oil
- 3 tablespoons chopped fresh cilantro
- 2 teaspoons sesame seeds, toasted (in dry skillet over medium heat for 3-5 minutes)

Direction

- Cook rice according to package directions.
- Meanwhile, combine sake and next 3 ingredients in large skillet deep enough to hold steamer rack. Bring liquid to boil. Reduce heat; simmer 5 minutes.
- Arrange fish on rack; sprinkle with salt and pepper. Place rack in skillet. Top fish with onions; drizzle with soy sauce and sesame oil.

Cover skillet; steam fish until opaque in center, about 5 minutes.

- Remove steamer rack.
- Mix cilantro into juices in skillet. Spoon rice onto plates.
- Top with fish, juices from skillet, and sesame seeds.
- Nutritional Info: Per serving: calories, 367; total fat, 5 g; saturated fat, 1 g; cholesterol, 62 mg; fiber, 1 g

256. Salmon And Corn Casserole Recipe

Serving: 6 | Prep: | Cook: 45mins | Ready in:

Ingredients

- 1 can (14-3/4 ounces) salmon, boned and skin removed
- milk
- 3 Tbs of butter
- 1/2 cup chopped onion
- 1/2 cup chopped green bell pepper
- 2 eggs, beaten
- 2 cups shredded sharp cheddar cheese
- 1 can 15 ounces) creamed corn
- 1/4 tps. salt
- 1/2 tps. pepper
- 1-1/4 cups crushed crackers

Direction

- Preheat the oven to 350 F.
- Drain the salmon, pouring the liquid into a glass measuring cup. Flake the salmon and place in a large mixing bowl. Add enough milk to the measuring cup to make 1 cup of liquid. Add to the salmon.
- Melt 2 Tbs. of the butter in a small skillet over medium heat. Add the onion and green pepper and sauté until limp, about 4 minutes. Add to the salmon, along with the eggs, cheese, corn, salt and pepper. Mix well. Spoon into a 9-inch by 13- inch baking dish.
- Melt the remaining 1 Tbs. butter and combine with the crushed crackers. Sprinkle over the top of the casserole. Bake for 45 minutes, uncovered. Serve hot.

257. Salmon Cakes Recipe

Serving: 4 | Prep: | Cook: 10mins | Ready in:

Ingredients

- 1 pound cooked fresh salmon or canned salmon
- T butter
- 1/4 cup finely chopped onion
- 2 tsp finely minced green pepper
- 1/2 cup finely minced celery
- 3/4 cup bread crumbs
- 1/4 cup finely chopped parsley
- 2 eggs, lightly beaten
- salt and ground black pepper to taste

Direction

- Flake the salmon in a bowl.
- Heat tablespoon of butter in a pan.
- Add the onion, celery and green pepper and cook until tender.
- Onion should be transparent.
- Cool mixture slightly and then add to salmon.
- Add the bread crumbs, parsley, eggs, salt, and pepper.
- Shape into 4 cakes.
- Chill for about 30 minutes.
- Heat some olive oil which should just be enough to cover bottom of a frying pan.
- Add the salmon cakes and cook until brown on both sides.
- Serve garnished with lemon wedges.
- Also recommend tartar sauce on the side.

258. Salmon Cannelloni With Lemon Cream Sauce Recipe

Serving: 6 | Prep: | Cook: 30mins | Ready in:

Ingredients

- For crespelle
- 2 large eggs
- 2/3 cup water
- 1/2 cup all-purpose flour
- 1/4 teaspoon salt
- 1 tablespoon finely chopped fresh tarragon
- 3 tablespoons unsalted butter, melted
- For sauce
- 2 tablespoons unsalted butter, cut into pieces
- 2 tablespoons all-purpose flour
- 1 (8-oz) bottle clam juice
- 1/3 cup water
- 1/4 cup heavy cream
- 2 teaspoons finely grated fresh lemon zest
- 1/4 teaspoon black pepper
- For salmon cannelloni
- 2 tablespoons unsalted butter, softened
- 1 shallot, finely chopped
- 1 teaspoon salt
- 1/2 teaspoon black pepper
- 6 (5-oz) center-cut pieces salmon fillet (preferably wild; 1 inch thick), skin and little bones discarded

Direction

- Make crespelle:
- Blend together eggs, water, flour, and salt in a blender until smooth. Transfer to a bowl and stir in tarragon.
- Lightly brush a 10-inch non-stick skillet with melted butter and heat over moderate heat until hot but not smoking. Ladle about 1/4 cup batter into skillet, tilting and rotating skillet to coat bottom, then pour excess batter back into bowl. (If batter sets before skillet is coated, reduce heat slightly for next crespella.) Cook until just set and underside is lightly browned, about 30 seconds, then invert crespella onto a clean kitchen towel in one layer to cool. (It will be cooked on one side only.) Make 5 more crespelle with remaining batter in same manner, brushing skillet with butter as needed and transferring to towel as cooked, arranging them in one layer.
- Make sauce:
- Heat butter in a 1- to 2-quart heavy saucepan over moderately low heat until foam subsides. Add flour and cook, whisking, 2 minutes. Add clam juice and water in a slow stream, whisking, then bring to a boil, whisking. Reduce heat and simmer, whisking occasionally, 5 minutes. Stir in cream, zest, and pepper, then remove from heat.
- Assemble cannelloni:
- Put oven rack in middle position and preheat oven to 425°F. Butter a 13- by 9-inch or other 3-quart glass or ceramic baking dish and spread half of sauce in dish.
- Stir together butter (2 tablespoons), shallot, salt, and pepper and spread 1 teaspoon on top of each fillet.
- Put 1 crespella, pale side down, on a work surface, then place 1 salmon fillet, buttered side down, in center of crespella and fold crespella around salmon, leaving ends open. Transfer to baking dish, arranging, seam side down, in sauce. Make 5 more cannelloni with remaining salmon and crespelle in same manner, arranging in baking dish. Spoon remaining sauce over cannelloni.
- Bake until salmon is just cooked through and sauce is bubbling, 15 to 20 minutes.
- Notes:
- • Sauce can be made 1 day ahead and cooled, uncovered, then chilled, covered. Thin with water if necessary.
- • Cannelloni can be assembled and covered with sauce (but not baked) 1 day ahead and chilled, wrapped tightly in plastic wrap. Bring to room temperature before baking.
- • Crespelle can be made 3 days ahead and chilled, wrapped tightly in plastic wrap.

259. Salmon Croquettes Recipe

Serving: 4 | Prep: | Cook: 20mins | Ready in:

Ingredients

- 2 Tablespoons light butter
- 5 Tablespoons flour
- 1 Cup canned salmon, cleaned
- 1/2 Cup milk
- 2 Large eggs, beaten
- 1 Cup bread Crumbs
- 1/3 Cup cracker crumbs
- 1 Can cream of mushroom soup or Ketchup (optional)
- cooking oil

Direction

- Clean the salmon, break it apart and remove any skin or gristle.
- Melt the butter, add flour and blend together. Stir in the milk gradually and cook 5 minutes over medium heat until the mixture is thick and smooth, stirring constantly.
- Add the salmon and 1 well beaten egg and bread crumbs. Mix thoroughly and chill for an hour in the refrigerator.
- Form the mixture into croquettes, dip in the other egg and roll in cracker crumbs.
- Pour about 1/4 inch of cooking oil and bring to medium high heat for frying. Fry croquettes for 3 to 5 minutes, turning to brown on all sides.
- Drain well on paper towels.
- Heat the soup for a sauce, or use ketchup.

260. Salmon Hobo Packs Recipe

Serving: 4 | Prep: | Cook: 12mins | Ready in:

Ingredients

- 2 lb. skinless salmon fillets, about 1-inch thick
- salt and freshly ground pepper
- 1/2 cup light-colored molasses
- 1/4 cup packed brown sugar
- 1 Tbsp. soy sauce
- 12 oz. green beans, or haricot verts (tender young green beans), ends trimmed
- 2 small yellow summer squash, halved lengthwise and cut into 1/2-inch slices
- 2 Tbsp. coarse grain mustard
- 2 Tbsp. snipped fresh parsley, optional
- 2 tsp. finely shredded lemon peel, optional
- 1/4 tsp. freshly ground pepper, optional

Direction

- Sprinkle salmon lightly with salt and pepper; set aside. For glaze, in a small saucepan stir together molasses, brown sugar, and soy sauce*; heat just until sugar is dissolved, stirring occasionally. Set aside.
- Grill salmon directly over medium coals for 6 minutes; turn. Grill for 4 minutes; brush with molasses mixture. Grill for 2 to 4 minutes more or until fish flakes easily with fork, brushing occasionally with glaze. Remove from grill. Cut salmon into 8 pieces. Cover and refrigerate 4 of the portions.
- Tear off four 36x18-inch sheets of heavy foil; fold in half to make 18-inch squares. In a bowl combine beans and squash; toss with mustard. Sprinkle lightly with salt and pepper. Divide evenly among foil sheets, placing vegetable mixture in the center. Place a salmon portion on each; spoon on any remaining glaze. Bring up two opposite edges of foil and seal with a double fold. Fold remaining edges together to completely enclose, leaving space for steam to build.
- Grill foil packets directly over medium coals for 20 minutes.
- To serve, transfer salmon and vegetables from packets to dinner plates. Combine parsley, lemon peel, and the 1/4 teaspoon pepper; sprinkle on salmon.

261. Salmon Lime Light Recipe

Serving: 2 | Prep: | Cook: 30mins | Ready in:

Ingredients

- 1 Tbl butter, not margerine
- 2 4 oz salmon fillets, skin removed
- 2 Tbl lime juice
- 1 Tbl teriyaki sauce
- 2 green onions, sliced (white part only)
- ½ tsp herbs de Provence
- 1 lime, cut into wedges (optional)

Direction

- 450 oven.
- Add butter to baking dish, melt, turn dish to coat.
- Place fillets in baking dish, unskinned side up.
- Stir together all ingredients except lime wedges.
- Drizzle over salmon.
- Bake until fish flakes easily with fork, about 25-30 minutes.
- Serve with lime wedges, if desired.

262. Salmon Patties Smothered In Creamed Peas Recipe

Serving: 2 | Prep: | Cook: 10mins | Ready in:

Ingredients

- salmon Patties
- 7 ounce can red salmon, drained, skin and bones removed (I know, I know…the bones are actually good for you, but I still like to pick out the big pieces!)
- ¼ cup diced onion
- 8 saltine crackers, finely crushed (I've also used finely crushed garlic croutons for a nice flavor enhancer)
- 1 egg, beaten
- ¼ teaspoon garlic salt
- 1/8 teaspoon Emeril's fish Rub (optional, but it's good stuff)
- 1/8 teaspoon pepper
- flour for coating salmon patties
- 2 tablespoons butter for frying pan
- Creamed peas
- 2 tablespoons butter (no margarine, please)
- 2 tablespoons flour
- ¼ teaspoon salt (I like to use sea salt, if I've got it on hand)
- 1/8 teaspoon Jane's Crazy Mixed Up Salt (optional, but pick some up if you've never tired it – it's a great seasoning, and I'm pretty sure it's available online, too)
- 1/8 teaspoon pepper
- 1 cup half-and-half (of course you can use milk, but I'm going for a richer sauce here!)
- 8.5 ounce can Le Sueur Very Young Small sweet peas (these make THE best creamed peas, but use whatever is available in your area), drained well

Direction

- It's best to make the creamed peas first, so it's ready to pour over the salmon patties when they are done – the patties take very little time to fry up.
- For the creamed peas, melt the butter in a small pan and stir in the flour and seasonings.
- Gradually stir in the half-and-half, using a whisk to help prevent lumps.
- Heat, whisking often, until sauce begins to thicken.
- Add drained peas and gently stir with a spoon (a whisk may break up the peas too much).
- Stir often as it continues to heat and thicken.
- To prepare the salmon patties, break up the salmon in a shallow bowl and mix with remaining patty ingredients.
- Sprinkle a piece of waxed paper generously with some flour.

- Shape salmon into 3 or 4 patties, and place them in the flour.
- Carefully flip the patties over so both sides are coated with the flour.
- Preheat skillet until hot (but not hot enough to burn the butter when added) and add butter to pan - as soon as it's melted, place the salmon patties into the hot, melted butter.
- Fry until golden on bottom, then carefully flip and continue to fry until brown on bottom.
- Serve immediately with creamed peas poured over each patty.

263. Salmon Souffle Recipe

Serving: 4 | Prep: | Cook: 45mins | Ready in:

Ingredients

- 1 small green bell pepper coarsely chopped
- 1 small red bell pepper coarsely chopped
- 1 tablespoon margarine
- 1/4 cup all purpose flour
- 1-1/2 cups milk
- 10 ounces frozen whole kernel corn
- 3/4 teaspoon dried dill weed
- 1/4 teaspoon salt
- 1/8 teaspoon white pepper
- 3 egg yolks lightly beaten
- 6-1/2 ounce can salmon drained flaked and bones removed
- 5 egg whites
- 1/8 teaspoon cream of tartar

Direction

- Sauté bell peppers in margarine for 5 minutes then stir in flour and cook 2 minutes.
- Gradually blend in milk, corn, dill weed, salt and pepper then heat to boiling over medium heat.
- Remove from heat.
- Gradually stir in small amount of vegetables into egg yolks then stir yolks into vegetables.
- Mix in salmon then beat egg whites and cream of tartar in large bowl to stiff peaks.
- Fold into salmon mixture then pour into lightly greased soufflé dish.
- Bake uncovered at 350 for 45 minutes then serve immediately.

264. Salmon Wellington Recipe

Serving: 8 | Prep: | Cook: 40mins | Ready in:

Ingredients

- 2 lb. skinned salmon side (up to 2 1/2 lb.)
- 1 package of defrosted puff pasty
- 1 egg beaten with a scant tablespoon of cream
- 3 tablespoons of butter
- 1 tablespoon of oil
- 2 leeks, cleaned and sliced thin as possible
- 2 packages of frozen artichoke hearts, defrosted and chopped
- 1 teaspoon of salt
- several grinds of black pepper
- 1 teaspoon of dried tarragon
- 1/4 to 1/2 cup of dry vermouth
- 1 1/2 cup prepared hollandaise sauce, with a very generous pinch of tarragon and parsley added. I generally increase the lemon juice to make it quite tart for a hollandaise.

Direction

- In a sauté pan, heat the oil and butter over medium heat.
- Add the leeks and sauté for a couple of minutes.
- Add the artichokes, seasonings, and vermouth.
- Cook until the liquid is nearly completely evaporated.
- Cool and reserve the filling.
- Preheat your oven to 400 degrees.
- Line a sheet pan with parchment paper.

- Roll out the puff pastry until it is as long as the side of salmon and at least 1 inch wider than the fish.
- Put on the prepped sheet pan.
- Place salmon on pastry. Top with the filling.
- Roll out the other piece of pastry, top the fish and filling.
- Seal the edges well.
- Brush with egg and cream.
- Bake at 400 degrees for 40 minutes until golden brown.
- Allow to rest for 10 minutes.
- Slice and serve with warm hollandaise sauce on the side.

265. Salmon With Basil Pesto And Polenta Crust Recipe

Serving: 6 | Prep: | Cook: 15mins | Ready in:

Ingredients

- 2 cups half-and-half
- 1/2 cup polenta (a.k.a. corn grits. I like Bob's Red Mill brand)
- 2 tablespoons mascarpone
- 1/4 tsp kosher salt
- 1/4 cup white wine
- 3 tablespoons unsalted butter
- Six 6-oz pieces of fresh salmon filet, each about 2 inches wide, seasoned on each side with kosher salt and pepper, skin on or off (I leave it on because it helps keep the salmon in one piece)
- 1/4 cup fresh basil pesto (recipe below)
- 2 tablespoons chopped Italian parsley
- ~~~~~~
- Fresh basil pesto Recipe:
- 2 cups fresh basil leaves, packed
- 1/2 cup freshly grated parmigiano-reggiano cheese (tip: grate it in your food processor before you start the pesto)
- 1/2 cup extra virgin olive oil
- 1/3 cup pine nuts
- 3 medium sized garlic cloves, minced
- salt and freshly ground black pepper to taste
- Combine the basil in with the pine nuts, pulse a few times in a food processor. Add the garlic, pulse a few times more.
- Slowly add the olive oil in a constant stream while the food processor is on. Stop to scrape down the sides of the food processor with a rubber spatula. Add the grated cheese and pulse again until blended. Add a pinch of salt and freshly ground black pepper to taste. Makes 1 cup.

Direction

- Preheat broiler. Bring the half-n-half to a boil in medium saucepan, and lower the heat to a simmer. Add salt and gradually add the polenta, whisking constantly until it is incorporated. Using a wooden spoon, continue cooking and string until mixture thickens, 3-4 minutes. Remove from heat and stir in mascarpone.
- Simmer the white wine in a small saucepan until reduced to about 3 tablespoons. Remove from heat, stir in lemon juice and butter, and keep warm.
- Broil salmon filets until cooked through, about 4 minutes per side (less if you like the center rare). Remove the salmon from the broiler and spread basil pesto over the tops. Spread the polenta evenly over the pesto and return to broiler to brown, 3-4 minutes.
- Stir fresh parsley into the lemon butter sauce and drizzle it around the fillets.
- Note: the polenta may be made up to 8 hours in advance and refrigerated until ready to use. Bring to room temp to make more malleable.

266. Salmon With Fried Capers Recipe

Serving: 4 | Prep: | Cook: 20mins | Ready in:

Ingredients

- 4 salmon steaks
- 1/2 teaspoon salt
- 1 teaspoon freshly ground black pepper
- 2 tablespoons grated lemon peel
- 3 tablespoons minced chives
- 5 tablespoons butter
- vegetable oil
- 2 tablespoons capers

Direction

- Preheat oven to 350.
- Pat fish dry with paper towels then sprinkle with salt and pepper and place in baking dish.
- Sprinkle with lemon peel and chives then dot with butter.
- Bake 12 minutes.
- While fish bakes put 1/2" oil in small saucepan set over high heat.
- Pat capers dry with paper towels.
- Add capers to hot oil and cook 2 minutes.
- Immediately remove with a slotted spoon to paper towels.
- Place fish on warm plates then divide cooking juices among them.
- Sprinkle with capers then serve immediately.

267. Salmon With Ginger Scallion Sauce Recipe

Serving: 2 | Prep: | Cook: 10mins | Ready in:

Ingredients

- 2 salmon fillets, Skin On thoroughly scaled, (Approx. 1 inch Thick)
- 1/4 Cup Fresh ginger (1/4 inch Dice)
- 4 scallions (Sliced on a bias 1 1/2 Inch Long)
- 3/4 Cup dry white wine
- 2 Tbls soy sauce
- 1/2 Cup water
- 1 Tsp sugar
- 1 - 2 Tables olive oil
- toasted sesame oil (Garnish)
- salt & pepper

Direction

- Place Fillets on paper towels and pat dry. Make sure both skin and flesh sides are very dry. Salt & Pepper both sides.
- Place a heavy 10 - 12 inch skillet on high heat. When hot, add Olive Oil to barely coat bottom.
- When oil smokes, place Salmon Fillets skin side down in skillet. Sear on high 1 min. Turn heat to Med High and cook 2 mins longer. (Do not move or touch the Fillets until you flip them)
- Flip Fillets and cook 2 mins. Remove to a rack and place flesh side down. Remove crispy skin (It will pull off easily) set aside for garnish.
- Turn heat back to high. Add Ginger. Cook 1 min. Add Scallions. Cook 30 sec. Add wine. Deglaze until the Wine reduces to 1/2 cup or less.
- Add Water, Soy Sauce, and Sugar. Bring to a simmer and reduce heat to med. Simmer approx. 1 - 2 Mins.
- Place Fillets back in the pan with the now skinned side down. Simmer for approx. 1 min. or to desired doneness.
- To Serve: Remove Salmon Fillets to a serving plate. Spoon the Ginger/Scallion sauce over the Salmon and drizzle with toasted Sesame Oil, Garnish with rolled up crispy skin and some chopped Scallion.
- This dish goes very well with Lemon or Orange-zested Jasmine Rice.

268. Salmon And Dill In Puff Pastry Recipe

Serving: 4 | Prep: | Cook: 20mins | Ready in:

Ingredients

- 8 oz fresh salmon
- or

- 1 large can salmon
- 4 oz sour cream
- 1 oz fresh chopped or 1 Tbsp dried dill
- 8 oz roll puff pastry
- 1 egg, beaten with 2 tsp water

Direction

- Preheat oven to 350F.
- Grease cookie tray or line with parchment paper.
- Roll out puff pastry 1/4 inch thick on a lightly floured board.
- Cut into 4 equal rectangles or cut into 4 fish shapes.
- Make 4 small rectangles with raised edges .
- Place rectangles or 2 fish shapes on baking tray and bake for 5 minutes until pastry begins to become firm.
- Remove from oven and layer with salmon.
- Mix dill and sour cream, then spread over salmon.
- If you are using fish shapes, place the 2 remaining fish shapes on top of the salmon and sour cream.
- Brush pastry with beaten egg and water mixture.
- Place in oven and bake for 15 minutes or until pastry is golden brown.
- Serve topped with a sprig or two of fresh dill.
- If you are not artistic with puff pastry, you can roll out the puff pastry into 4 squares and make a simple salmon wrap to bake. Be sure to seal the edges and brush with egg mixture.

269. Salmon And Leeks Recipe

Serving: 4 | Prep: | Cook: 20mins | Ready in:

Ingredients

- 1/2 cup butter
- 4 salmon fillets
- 2 leeks finely sliced
- 1/2 cup white wine
- 1/4 cup olive oil
- 2 tablespoons finely chopped chervil
- 1 tablespoon fresh lemon juice

Direction

- Preheat oven to 350 then smear 4 large circles of parchment paper with butter.
- Place a salmon fillet in center of each one and top with 1/4 of the leeks.
- Divide olive oil, wine and chervil among each and season well.
- Draw up edges of the paper and fold edges to make packets.
- Place on baking sheet and cook 20 minutes.
- Open packets carefully and keep juices and leeks with salmon as you serve it with lemon juice.

270. Salmon And Noodles Recipe

Serving: 2 | Prep: | Cook: 30mins | Ready in:

Ingredients

- 2 tablespoons butter
- 1/2 cup chopped white onion
- 1/4 cup green pepper chopped
- 2 cups medium egg noodles cooked and drained
- 1 can condensed cream of mushroom soup
- 1 cup salmon drained and flaked
- 1/4 cup shredded cheddar cheese

Direction

- Cook onion and green pepper in butter until soft.
- Combine with noodles, soup and salmon.
- Place in casserole dish and top with cheese.
- Bake at 400 for 30 minutes.

271. Salmon And Peas With Vegetable Spaghetti Squash Recipe

Serving: 3 | Prep: | Cook: 5mins | Ready in:

Ingredients

- 1 tbsp reduced sodium soy sauce
- 1 tbsp honey
- 2 tbsp water
- 1 tsp ground ginger
- 1 tsp cornstarch
- 2 slices of sweet onion diced
- 1 1/3 cups frozen peas
- 8oz salmon fillet cut in strips
- 2 cups cooked spaghetti squash
- salt and pepper to preference

Direction

- Whisk the soy sauce, honey, water, ginger and cornstarch.
- Set aside.
- Heat a skillet over medium setting.
- Warm the onion and add the frozen peas.
- Cook for a minute or two allowing the peas to defrost.
- Add the salmon and cook for 3-4 minutes only stirring about every minute.
- If you stir more, the salmon will break up too much.
- After the 4 minutes pour the soy sauce mixture over, stir in and cook for one minute.
- It will thicken and coat everything.
- Separate into two servings and scoop over warm spaghetti squash.

272. Salmon In Phyllo Pastry With Mango Curry Sauce Recipe

Serving: 4 | Prep: | Cook: 25mins | Ready in:

Ingredients

- 4 pieces of fresh salmon filet (about 1 lb)
- 16 pieces of phyllo pastry sheets
- 1 stick melted butter or margarine
- mango curry sauce:
- 1 large ripe mango, coarse chopped
- 1/2 cup mayonnaise, maybe a bit more if desired
- 2 tsp curry powder or to taste
- 1/2 cup toasted chopped walnuts (optional)

Direction

- Make the mango curry sauce by combining ingredients and chill well.
- To prepare salmon: salt and pepper pieces.
- Lay 2 sheets of phyllo on flat surface and brush with melted butter.
- Add 2 more sheets and brush with melted butter.
- Place 1/4 of mango mixture in middle of phyllo several inches up from bottom edge.
- Place on salmon. Fold (roll) phyllo over salmon and tuck under edges.
- Repeat for 3 more servings.
- Place salmon pastries into a buttered baking pan and brush tops of pastry with more melted butter.
- Bake 400F about 25 minutes or until pastry is golden.
- Makes 4 main dish servings or cut each in half for 8 appetizers servings

273. Salmon To Die For Recipe

Serving: 3 | Prep: | Cook: 6mins | Ready in:

Ingredients

- 1 large fresh filet of salmon about eight inches long
- capers
- dash kosher salt
- fresh ground pepper
- 4 tbls white 'drinking wine' (serve with if so inclined)
- wax paper

Direction

- Gently wash fish and feel for any bones
- Pat dry
- Place skin down in middle of wax paper
- Add salt pepper and wine
- Fold paper till sides meet on top and fold over to close on top leaving air space between fish and 'roof' of paper
- Fold and enclose both ends
- Place in micro for 6 minutes

274. Salmon With Garden Sauce Recipe

Serving: 4 | Prep: | Cook: 10mins | Ready in:

Ingredients

- 1 cup fresh parsley leaves
- 2 cups fresh spinach leaves, well washed
- 1/2 cup mayo
- 1/3 cup sour cream
- 1 Tbls fresh lemon juice
- 3/4 ts salt, divided
- 4 salmon steaks, 6 ounces each and about 3/4" thick

Direction

- Bring a medium sauce pan of water to a rapid boil over high heat
- Plunge spinach leaves into water just until wilted, approx. 10 secs.
- Rinse under cold running water and drain well.
- Transfer spinach and parsley to a blender or food processor.
- Add the mayo, sour cream, lemon juice and 1/4 tsp. salt to the mixture in the blender.
- Blend or process until smooth.
- Chill for at least 30 minutes up to 12 hours
- Preheat broiler.
- Sprinkle the salmon steaks with the remainder of salt.
- Place on broiler pan and broil 6" from heat, turning once just until cooked through, approx. 8 minutes.
- Transfer to serving plate and spoon the sauce over the salmon steaks or could serve the sauce on the side depending on preferences.

275. Salmon With Sesame Ginger Glaze Recipe

Serving: 4 | Prep: | Cook: 10mins | Ready in:

Ingredients

- ¼ c packed brown sugar
- 2 Tbsp Dijon mustard
- 1 Tbsp grated fresh or 1 tsp ground ginger
- 1 Tbsp sesame seeds
- 4 6-oz wild Pacific salmon fillets, about 1" thick, skinned
- ½ tsp salt
- ½ tsp freshly ground black pepper

Direction

- 1. Coat rack of baking sheet with cooking spray. Preheat broiler.
- 2. In small bowl, combine sugar, mustard, sesame seeds and ginger. Season both sides of fillets with salt and pepper. Place salmon on broiler rack and brush glaze on top. Broil (6" from heat) 8 to 10 minutes or until fish is lightly browned.

276. Salt Cod In Olive And Tomatoe Confit Recipe

Serving: 6 | Prep: | Cook: 30mins | Ready in:

Ingredients

- 1.5 lb skinless boneless salt cod (bacalao)
- 8 large garlic cloves, minced
- 1/3 c olive oil
- 2 (14-oz) cans diced tomatoes, drained
- 1/2 c green olives, sliced
- 1 bay leaf
- 1/4 tsp sugar
- 6 tbsp mayonnaise
- 1/4 c crème fraîche
- 1 tbsp water

Direction

- Cover cod with 2 inches of cold water in a large bowl and soak in the fridge, changing water 3 times a day for 2 to 3 days.
- Drain cod and transfer to a 3-quart saucepan, then add 6 cups water. If fish is large, cut into 4 to 6 oz. portions.
- Bring cod to a gentle simmer and remove from heat.
- Gently transfer cod with a slotted spatula to a paper-towel-lined plate to drain.
- Cover with a dampened paper towel and chill while making confit.
- Cook garlic in oil in a skillet over moderately low heat, turning occasionally, until golden.
- Add tomatoes, bay leaf and sugar and cook until tomatoes thickens, and breaks down into a very thick sauce.
- Add salt and pepper to taste.
- Fish out bay leaf.
- Spread sauce in a large baking dish and arrange fish over sauce.
- Sprinkle green olives on top.
- Whisk together mayonnaise, crème fraiche, and water and spread over each piece of fish.
- Broil fish 5 to 6 inches from heat just until mayonnaise mixture is lightly browned approx. 2 minutes.

277. Saumon Aux Lentilles Salmon With Lentils And Mustard Herb Butter Recipe

Serving: 4 | Prep: | Cook: 40mins | Ready in:

Ingredients

- For mustard-Herb Butter:
- 5 tablespoons unsalted butter, softened
- 1 tablespoon chopped chives
- 1 teaspoon chopped tarragon
- 2 teaspoons grainy mustard
- 2 teaspoons fresh lemon juice
- ~~~~
- For Lentils:
- 1 cup French green lentils
- 4 cups water
- 2 medium leeks (white and pale green parts only)
- 1 tablespoon unsalted butter
- 1/2 to 1 tablespoon fresh lemon juice
- ~~~~
- For Salmon:
- 4 (6-ounce) pieces skinless salmon fillet
- 2 tablespoons unsalted butter

Direction

- Make Mustard-Herb Butter:
- Stir together all ingredients with 1/4 teaspoon each of salt and pepper.
- ~~~~
- Cook Lentils:
- Bring lentils, water, and 3/4 teaspoon salt to a boil in a heavy medium saucepan, then reduce heat and simmer, uncovered, until lentils are just tender, 20 to 25 minutes.
- Remove from heat and let stand 5 minutes.

- Reserve 1/2 cup cooking liquid, then drain lentils.
- ~~~~
- While lentils cook, chop leeks, and then wash. Cook leeks in butter in a heavy medium skillet over medium-low heat, stirring occasionally, until softened, 6 to 8 minutes.
- Add lentils with reserved cooking liquid to leeks along with 3 tablespoons mustard-herb butter and cook, stirring, until lentils are heated through and butter is melted.
- Add lemon juice and salt and pepper to taste.
- Remove from heat and keep warm, covered.
- ~~~~
- Sauté Salmon While Leeks Cook:
- Pat salmon dry and sprinkle with 1/2 teaspoon salt and 1/4 teaspoon pepper (total).
- Heat butter in a large non-stick skillet over medium-high heat until foam subsides, then sauté salmon, turning once, until golden and just cooked through, 6 to 8 minutes total.
- Serve salmon, topped with remaining mustard-herb butter, over lentils.
- ~~~~
- NOTES:
- ~ Mustard-herb butter can be made 1 day ahead and chilled, covered. Soften at room temperature before using (1 hour).
- ~ Lentils can be cooked (but not drained) 1 day ahead and chilled in cooking liquid, covered (once cool).

278. Savory Salmon Recipe

Serving: 4 | Prep: | Cook: 27mins | Ready in:

Ingredients

- 1 (2-pound) salmon fillet
- House seasoning, recipe follows
- 1 small red bell pepper, julienne
- 1 small green bell pepper, julienne
- 1 medium onion, sliced thin
- 1 medium orange, sectioned and seeded
- 1 pint strawberries, cleaned and sliced
- 1/2 cup water
- 1/2 cup honey
- 1/2 cup chopped fresh chervil or baby dill
- 4 cloves garlic, minced
- 2 tablespoons chopped green onion
- 2 lemons, juiced
- House Seasoning:
- 1 cup salt
- 1/4 cup black pepper
- 1/4 cup garlic powder
- Mix well. Store in shaker near stove for convenience.

Direction

- Preheat oven to 350 degrees F.
- Place salmon fillet on a foil-lined pan. Season with House Seasoning, then cover and surround fish with red and green bell pepper, onion, and sectioned orange slices. Mix strawberries, water, honey, chervil or dill, garlic and green onions together. Pour lemon juice over salmon. Ladle strawberry mixture evenly over salmon. Cover with foil and pierce foil, allowing steam to escape. Bake for 25 to 30 minutes. Serve with rice.

279. Sea Bass With Ratatouille Jus And Roasted Lemon Asparagus Recipe

Serving: 4 | Prep: | Cook: 75mins | Ready in:

Ingredients

- 1½ lb sea bass fillet, about 1 inch thick, cut into 4pieces
- olive oil
- basil
- salt and pepper
- Ratatouille Jus:
- 1 large onion, thinly sliced
- 2 red peppers, cored and thinly sliced

- 2 garlic cloves, smashed
- 2 small zucchini, cut in half and thinly sliced
- 2 small yellow squash, cut in half and thinly sliced
- olive oil
- red wine vinegar
- Tabasco .
- salt and pepper
- roasted lemon Asparagus:
- 2 Tbsp fresh lemon juice
- 1 Tbsp extra-virgin olive oil
- 1 tsp finely grated lemon zest
- 12 asparagus spears, peeled and trimmed
- salt and pepper

Direction

- For the Ratatouille Jus
- Add olive oil to a sauté pan over medium heat. Add all the sliced vegetables and garlic.
- Cook for 3-5 minutes - do not brown. Add salt and pepper.
- At this point, I generally pull out about 3 slices of zucchini, 3 slices of yellow squash, and 4 slices of red pepper. I will keep these vegetables cool until I am ready to plate the fish. Then I finely dice the reserved vegetables and use them as a garnish just before serving. This is entirely up to you, but it does make a much better presentation, and adds a bit of crunch.
- Reduce heat and cook remaining vegetables slowly for 1 hour. Add a touch of water if necessary (though I've never felt the need to add any water).
- Place cooked vegetables in a blender with a touch of water at the bottom of blender.
- Blend, adjust seasoning, and allow to cool.
- Once the mixture has cooled, add a touch vinegar and Tabasco and check seasoning again. The sauce should have a nice consistency, not too thick and not runny.
- For the Roasted Asparagus
- Preheat oven to 450° F.
- Mix lemon juice, oil, and lemon zest in a small bowl.
- Place asparagus in a larger bowl and pour in sauce. Sprinkle with salt and pepper and toss.
- Place asparagus on a baking sheet.
- Roast asparagus until crisp-tender, turning occasionally, about 8 to 12 minutes.
- To Serve:
- Brush fish with olive oil and season with salt and pepper.
- Heat 2 Tbsp olive oil in a skillet, add fish fillets carefully, and sauté 3-4 minutes on each side, flipping very gently after the first 3-4 minutes (being careful not to break up the fillets).
- Squeeze lemon juice over fish.
- Pour a small amount of ratatouille jus on the plate to form a circle, lay one fish fillet on top of the jus, and arrange asparagus. If you like, spoon a bit more ratatouille jus over the fish before arranging the asparagus.
- Garnish with basil leaves and (if you've reserved any of the vegetables) a bit of the finely diced squash, zucchini, and red pepper.

280. Sea Bass In Salt Crust Recipe

Serving: 4 | Prep: | Cook: 40mins | Ready in:

Ingredients

- 1 sea bass, about 2.2 lb cleaned and scaled
- 1 sprig each of fresh fennel, rosemary, and thyme
- Mixed peppercorns
- 4.5 lb coarse sea salt

Direction

- Preheat the oven to 475°F. Fill the cavity of the fish with the sprigs of fresh fennel, rosemary, and thyme, and grind over some of the mixed peppercorns.
- Spread half the salt on a shallow cookie sheet (ideally oval) and lay the sea bass on it. Cover the fish all over with a 1/2 inch layer of salt, pressing it down firmly. Moisten the salt

lightly by spraying with water from an atomizer. Bake the fish for 30-40 minutes, until the salt crust is just beginning to color.

- Bring the sea bass to the table in its salt crust. Use a sharp knife to break open the crust and cut into four portions.
- Serve.

281. Seafood Sauce For Shrimp Lobster Crab Or Salmon Recipe

Serving: 4 | Prep: | Cook: 30mins | Ready in:

Ingredients

- seafood Newburg Sauce (Serve with shrimp, lobster, crab or salmon over hot rice)
- 2 tablespoons butter
- 2 teaspoons shallots, minced, or finely minced onion
- 2 tablespoons paprika
- dry sherry to taste
- 2 tablespoons tomato paste
- 2 teaspoons brandy or dry sherry
- 2 cups cream sauce or white sauce (See Below)
- 1/8 teaspoon dried thyme
- pinch cayenne pepper
- 2 cups to 2 lbs hot seafood
- 3 cups - hot rice

Direction

- Melt butter in sauté pan. Add the shallots or onion and sauté over medium-low heat for 2 to 3 minutes, until translucent. Add the paprika and sherry, and sauté for 2 minutes longer. Stir in the tomato paste.
- Add the brandy or sherry to the sauté pan and cook a few minutes longer. Add the cream sauce, thyme, and cayenne. Cook for 2 minutes more.
- Makes about 2 1/2 cups.
- Cream Sauce
- 1/4 cup butter
- 1/4 cup flour
- 2 cups light cream
- 2 onions, studded with 3 cloves
- 2 bay leaves
- Salt and pepper -- to taste
- Fresh nutmeg, grated -- to taste
- Melt the butter in a saucepan over low heat. Stir in the flour, and cook, stirring, for 3 to 4 minutes; do not brown.
- In another saucepan, bring the cream just to a boil. Stir the warm cream into the flour mixture, whisking until smooth.
- Add the onions and bay leaves, and simmer for 20 minutes on low heat. Season sauce with salt, pepper and nutmeg. Strain the sauce and serve. Makes 2 cups.

282. Seafood Stuffed Flounder Recipe

Serving: 6 | Prep: | Cook: 30mins | Ready in:

Ingredients

- 2 lbs. skinless flounder 1/4 - 1/2 inch thick(can also use sole)
- 1 lb. sea scallops (can also use peeled cooked shrimp)
- 1 10 oz. pkg frozen chopped spinach, thawed
- 1 tbls. butter
- 1 onion, chopped
- 1 cup herb stuffing mix
- 1/2 cup sour cream
- 1/4 cup parmesan cheese
- 1 egg, lightly beaten

Direction

- Rinse fish and pat dry
- Cook scallops in boiling water 1-3 minutes or until scallops turn opaque
- Drain and cut into quarters
- Cook onion in butter until tender

- Squeeze water out of spinach
- Slightly crush stuffing mix
- In a mixing bowl, mix together onion, spinach, stuffing mix, sour cream, parmesan cheese, and egg.
- Carefully stir in scallops
- Preheat oven to 375
- Measuring length of fish to 6-7 inches, (overlap thinner ends of short fillets to make one)
- Spread about 1/2 cup of scallop mixture on top of each piece of fish
- Roll fish up starting at thin end and secure with a toothpick
- Bake for 20-25 minutes in a greased baking dish

283. Seared Salmon With Cilantro Cucumber Salsa Recipe

Serving: 4 | Prep: | Cook: 20mins | Ready in:

Ingredients

- 1/2 cucumber, peeled, halved, lengthwise, seeded, halved lengthwise again, and thinly sliced crosswise
- 1 cup cherry tomatoes, quartered
- 1/2 yellow or orange bell pepper, seeded and cut into 1-inch julienne3
- 2 Tablespoons chopped shallot or red onion
- 1 Tablespoon chopped fresh cilantro (fresh coriander) plus sprigs for garnish
- 1 Tablespoon lime juice
- 1-1/2 teaspoons canola oil
- 1 teaspoon honey
- 1/2 teaspoon red pepper flakes
- 1 teaspoon salt
- 4 salmon fillets, each 5 oz., about 1 inch thick
- 1/4 teaspoon freshly ground black pepper
- lime wedges for garnish

Direction

- In a bowl, combine the cucumber, tomatoes, bell pepper, shallot, and chopped cilantro. Toss gently to mix.
- In a small bowl, whisk together the lime juice, 1 teaspoon of the canola oil, the honey, red pepper flakes, and 1/2 teaspoon of the salt. Pour the lime mixture over the cucumber mixture and toss gently to mix and coat evenly. Set aside.
- Sprinkle the salmon fillets on both sides with the remaining 1/2 teaspoon salt and the black pepper. In a large non-stick frying pan, heat the remaining ½ teaspoon canola oil over medium-high heat.
- Add the fish to the pan and cook, turning once, until opaque throughout when tested with the tip of a knife, 4-5 minutes on each side.
- Transfer the salmon fillets to warmed individual plates and top each with one-fourth of the salsa. Garnish the plates with the cilantro sprigs and lime wedges. Serve immediately.

284. Seared Tuna Steaks With Wasabi Green Onion Mayonnaise Recipe

Serving: 4 | Prep: | Cook: 10mins | Ready in:

Ingredients

- 1/2 cup mayonnaise
- 2 tablespoons minced green onions (white and green parts)
- 1 teaspoon (or more) wasabi paste
- 2 tablespoons teriyaki sauce
- 1 tablespoon soy sauce
- 1 tablespoon unseasoned rice vinegar
- 4 8-ounce tuna steaks (preferably ahi; each about 1 inch thick)
- vegetable oil

Direction

- Whisk first 3 ingredients in small bowl to blend, adding more wasabi paste if desired. Cover and refrigerate.
- Whisk teriyaki sauce, soy sauce, and rice vinegar in small bowl to blend.
- Place tuna steaks in resealable plastic bag. Add teriyaki mixture; seal bag. Turn bag to coat. Let stand at room temperature 30 minutes, turning bag occasionally.
- Brush grill with vegetable oil.
- Prepare grill (medium-high heat).
- Drain tuna steaks. Grill tuna to desired doneness, about 4 minutes per side for medium.
- Top each tuna steak with about 2 tablespoons wasabi mayonnaise and serve.

285. Sesame Crusted Tilapia Recipe

Serving: 6 | Prep: | Cook: 15mins | Ready in:

Ingredients

- 2 lbs tilapia fillets
- 1 1/2 cups Asian Sesame dressing
- 1 cup panko
- 1/3 cup sesame seeds
- 1 teaspoon garlic powder
- 1 teaspoon ground ginger
- 1/2 teaspoon salt
- 1/4 teaspoon black pepper
- nonstick cooking spray

Direction

- Preheat oven to 375.
- Put foil on rimmed baking sheet and spray with nonstick cooking spray.
- Place Asian dressing in a shallow dish.
- In another shallow dish, combine Panko, sesame seeds, garlic powder, ginger, salt and pepper.
- Mix well.
- Dip fish lightly in dressing then into Panko mixture coating completely.
- Place on baking sheet.
- Lightly coat fish with cooking spray.
- Bake 10 to 15 minutes, or until fish flakes easily with a fork.
- Depending on the thickness of the fish, cooking times may vary.

286. Sesame Crusted Tuna With Asian Dipping Sauce Recipe

Serving: 46 | Prep: | Cook: 6mins | Ready in:

Ingredients

- 1 tablespoon chopped green onions
- 2 tablespoons low-sodium soy sauce
- 2 tablespoons fresh orange juice
- 1 tablespoon rice vinegar
- 1 teaspoon brown sugar
- 1 teaspoon grated lemon rind
- 2 teaspoons fresh lemon juice
- 2 teaspoons honey
- 1 1/4 teaspoons prepared wasabi paste
- 1 teaspoon grated peeled fresh ginger
- 2 teaspoons vegetable oil
- 4 (6-ounce) tuna steaks (about 3/4 inch thick)
- 1/4 teaspoon salt
- 3 tablespoons sesame seeds
- 2 tablespoons black sesame seeds
- Sliced green onions (optional)

Direction

- ****** DIPPING SAUCE *****
- Combine first 10 ingredients, stirring with a whisk.
- ****** SEARED TUNA *****
- Heat oil in a large non-stick skillet over medium-high heat.
- Sprinkle tuna with salt.
- Combine sesame seeds in a shallow dish.

- Lightly coat Tuna in Soy sauce.
- Dredge tuna in sesame seeds.
- Add tuna to pan; cook 3 minutes on each side or until desired degree of doneness.
- Garnish with green onions, if desired. Serve with that amazing dipping sauce.
- Try to contain yourself!!!

287. Simply Simple Salmon Cakes Recipe

Serving: 4 | Prep: | Cook: 15mins | Ready in:

Ingredients

- 1-2 lbs fresh or frozen salmon
- 1/2 large sweet onion
- bread crumbs (homemade are best -made from enriched bread and seasoned to your liking)
- eggs or eggbeaters
- oil and butter for frying
- =======
- frozen artichoke hearts
- grape tomatoes
- sliced sweet onion

Direction

- Place salmon in blender with onion
- Remove to bowl
- Add bread crumbs until the right consistency
- Using a small kitchen scale, make 4 -5 oz. patties
- Dip in egg
- Dip in breadcrumbs
- Place covered in fridge for at least an hour
- Place oil in pan
- Add artichokes, tomatoes and onion
- Fry on med to med high heat
- Add patties till crispy on outside
- That's it....enjoy!

288. Skillet Fillets With Cilantro Butter Recipe

Serving: 4 | Prep: | Cook: 6mins | Ready in:

Ingredients

- 1/4 teaspoon salt
- 1/4 teaspoon ground cumin
- 1/8 teaspoon ground red pepper
- 4 (6-ounce) tilapia fillets
- cooking spray
- 1 lemon, quartered
- 2 tablespoons butter, softened
- 2 tablespoons finely chopped fresh cilantro
- 1/2 teaspoon grated lemon rind
- 1/4 teaspoon paprika
- 1/8 teaspoon salt

Direction

- Combine first 3 ingredients; sprinkle over both sides of fish. Heat a large nonstick skillet over medium-high heat. Coat pan with cooking spray. Coat both sides of fish with cooking spray; place in pan. Cook 3 minutes on each side or until fish flakes easily when tested with a fork or until desired degree of doneness. Place fish on a serving platter; squeeze lemon quarters over fish.
- Place butter and remaining ingredients in a small bowl; stir until well blended. Serve with fish.

289. Slow Cooker Halibut Recipe

Serving: 4 | Prep: | Cook: 150mins | Ready in:

Ingredients

- 2 packages (12 oz. each) frozen halibut steaks, thawed
- 2 Tbs flour
- 1 Tbs sugar

- 1/2 tsp salt
- 1/4 cup butter
- 1/3 cup dry white wine
- 2/3 cup milk
- lemon wedges

Direction

- Pat the halibut steaks dry and place them in the slow cooker.
- In a small bowl, combine the flour, sugar and salt. In a sauce pan, melt the butter, and stir in the flour mixture.
- When well blended, add the wine and milk and cook over a medium heat until thickened, stirring constantly.
- Allow the sauce to boil for 1 minute while stirring.
- Pour the sauce over the fish.
- Cover and cook on High for 2 1/2 to 3 hours.
- Garnish with lemon wedges.

290. Slow Cooker Halibut In White Sauce Recipe

Serving: 6 | Prep: | Cook: 180mins |Ready in:

Ingredients

- 2 (12 oz) packages frozen halibut steaks, thawed
- 2 tbsp flour
- 1 tbsp sugar
- 1/4 tsp salt
- 1/4 c butter
- 1/3 c dry white wine
- 2/3 c milk

Direction

- Place halibut steaks in crock pot. Combine flour, sugar and salt. Melt the butter in a saucepan. Add the flour mixture, stir until bubbles. Add the wine and milk and boil for 1 minute or until thickened. Pour the sauce over the fish and cook on High for 3 hours.

291. Smoked Haddock And Cucumber Salad Recipe

Serving: 2 | Prep: | Cook: 10mins |Ready in:

Ingredients

- 1 pound smoked haddock fillets skinned and sliced
- 1/2 cucumber cut into strips
- 4 spring onions chopped
- Rind and juice of 1 lime
- 1 tablespoon fresh chopped chives
- 1 teaspoon salt
- 1 teaspoon freshly ground black pepper
- 4 ounces natural yogurt

Direction

- Place fish in a suitable container then add 2 tablespoons water.
- Cover and cook in microwave on high for 2 minutes.
- Remove fish slices using a slotted spoon and leave to cool.
- Mix together the cucumber and spring onion then arrange in a pile on a plate.
- Mix together the yogurt, chives, lime rind and juice.
- Place fish on top of cucumber mixture and pour over yogurt mixture.

292. Smoked Haddock And Zucchini Lasagne Recipe

Serving: 4 | Prep: | Cook: 25mins |Ready in:

Ingredients

- 3/4 pint (15 fl. oz.) milk
- 12 oz. smoked haddock fillet. The important thing is to use real peat-smoked haddock (which isn't a very deep colour), and avoid the orange-dyed stuff that some fishmongers try to pass off as the real thing. It will just give you an allergic reaction to the food colour and the other additives. Actually I reckon you could use any suitable flaky smoked fish of your choice, as long as it's not artificially coloured.
- 1 oz. butter
- 6 oz. courgettes (zucchini), sliced
- 4 oz. onions, chopped
- 1 heaped teaspoon chopped fresh tarragon
- Another 1 1/2 oz. butter
- 1 1/4 oz. plain flour
- About 8 oz. dried lasagne sheets
- 4 oz. grated cheese

Direction

- Preheat oven to Gas 4 180C/350F.
- In a pan, put the fish and the milk.
- Bring to a very low simmer.
- Cook the fish through, lightly - about 7 minutes or thereabouts, depending on how thick the fillets are.
- Remove the fish from the milk and reserve the milk.
- In a frying pan, heat the 1 oz. butter.
- Add the courgettes (zucchini), the onions and the tarragon.
- Sauté but do not color. Drain.
- In a heavy saucepan, heat the 1 1/2 oz. butter.
- Blend in the flour. Cook a little but do not allow to color.
- Then gradually, but quickly, blend in the milk in which the fish was cooked.
- Bring to the boil and cook over a gentle heat for 15 minutes. Check the seasoning.
- Butter a 10 x 8" baking dish.
- Spread some sauce over the bottom.
- On top, put a layer of lasagne.
- Cover with half the courgette/onion mixture and half the fish, flaked.
- Top with some more sauce.
- Another layer of lasagne.
- The other half of the fish, courgette and onion.
- Some more sauce.
- Another layer of lasagne.
- The last of the sauce.
- Scatter the cheese over the top.
- Bake for 25 minutes.

293. Smoked Salmon And Mozzarella Calzone Recipe

Serving: 4 | Prep: | Cook: 45mins | Ready in:

Ingredients

- Basic pizza dough
- 1/2 pound roma tomatoes, coarsely chopped (about 3 to 4 tomatoes)
- 1 teaspoon kosher salt
- 1 large egg
- 1 large egg yolk
- 1 teaspoon water
- 4 ounces cold-smoked salmon, thinly sliced
- 4 ounces fresh mozzarella, thinly sliced

Direction

- Prepare Basic Pizza Dough or you can buy premade. Keep at room temperature.
- Position rack in center of oven, and place a baking sheet on it. Heat oven to 400°F. Combine chopped tomatoes with salt, place in a colander or strainer set over a bowl, and let sit 20 minutes to drain.
- In a small bowl, whisk together egg, egg yolk, water, and a large pinch of salt until smooth; set aside.
- Divide pizza dough into 4 pieces. On a lightly floured surface, roll each piece into a paper-thin round, about 12 inches in diameter.
- Place 1/4 of the sliced salmon on the bottom left side of each dough round, about 1 inch from the edge. Top with 1/4 of the drained tomatoes, followed by 1/4 of the mozzarella. Brush the 1-inch-wide border of each dough

round with egg mixture, then fold each dough round in half and then fold in half again (it will resemble a quarter-circle shape).

- Using a fork, crimp the edges of each calzone to seal in the filling, and trim any excess dough so the edges are even. Brush the top of each calzone and the edges with egg mixture, place on the heated baking sheet, and bake until golden brown and puffed around the edges, about 20 minutes. Serve immediately.

294. Smoked Salmon Chowder Recipe

Serving: 6 | Prep: | Cook: 30mins | Ready in:

Ingredients

- 1/4 cup margarine
- 2 tablespoons bacon fat
- 1 small white onion diced
- 1/2 cup diced celery
- 3/4 pound red potatoes scrubbed and diced
- 1-1/2 teaspoons minced garlic
- 3/4 teaspoon dried thyme
- 1-1/2 teaspoons dried tarragon
- 3/4 teaspoon dried dill weed
- 1/2 cup all purpose flour
- 1-1/2 teaspoons paprika
- 7 cups fish stock
- 6 ounces smoked salmon diced
- 1 dried bay leaf
- 1 tablespoon lemon juice
- 1-1/2 teaspoons worcestershire sauce
- 1/8 teaspoon Tabasco sauce
- 3/4 teaspoon freshly ground black pepper
- 2 teaspoons salt
- 1/4 cup dry white wine
- 1 cup half-and-half
- 1/4 cup chopped fresh parsley

Direction

- In 4 quart pot melt margarine and bacon fat.
- Sauté onion, celery, potatoes, garlic, thyme, tarragon and dill over medium heat.
- When onions are translucent reduce heat and add flour and paprika blending well.
- Stir in stock then add salmon, bay leaf, juice, Worcestershire, Tabasco, salt, pepper and wine.
- Bring to a boil then reduce heat and simmer 20 minutes.
- Remove from heat and stir in half-and-half and parsley.
- Remove bay leaf before serving.

295. Smoked Salmon Cream Pasta Sauce Recipe

Serving: 4 | Prep: | Cook: 20mins | Ready in:

Ingredients

- 8 ounces smoked salmon
- 8 ounces heavy cream
- 1 teaspoon freshly ground black pepper
- 1 tablespoon chopped fresh dill
- dill for garnishing
- 16 ounces uncooked angel hair pasta

Direction

- Cook pasta according to package directions.
- Slice salmon into thin strips.
- Heat cream over low heat until bubbly and thick.
- Combine with cooked pasta over medium heat then add salmon and chopped dill.
- Mix well and serve garnished with fresh dill sprigs.

296. Smoked Trout Cakes With Horseradish Cream Recipe

Serving: 4 | Prep: | Cook: 10mins | Ready in:

Ingredients

- 1-1/2 cups flaked smoked trout
- 2 tablespoons chopped green onion
- 2 teaspoons capers drained and coarsely chopped
- 1/2 teaspoon grated lemon peel
- 1/4 teaspoon freshly ground pepper
- 1/4 teaspoon salt
- 1 large egg lightly beaten
- 1/4 cup whipping cream
- 1 cup fresh bread crumbs from French bread divided
- 3 tablespoons vegetable oil
- horseradish Cream:
- 1 cup sour cream
- 2 tablespoons grated fresh or prepared horseradish
- 1/8 teaspoon paprika
- 1 clove garlic minced
- 1/4 teaspoon salt
- 1/2 teaspoon freshly ground black pepper

Direction

- Combine trout, onion, capers, lemon peel and pepper in medium bowl then season with salt.
- Stir in egg, cream and 1/2 cup bread crumbs to blend.
- Form mixture by 1/4 cupfuls into eight 1/2" thick cakes.
- Place remaining breadcrumbs in shallow dish then roll cakes in breadcrumbs coating completely.
- Heat 2 tablespoons oil in large skillet over medium heat.
- Working in batches cook fish cakes until golden brown about 3 minutes per side.
- Add more oil as necessary then serve with horseradish cream.
- To make horseradish cream combine sour cream, horseradish, paprika and garlic until blended.
- Season with salt and pepper.

297. Snapper Pontchartrain Recipe

Serving: 4 | Prep: | Cook: 10mins | Ready in:

Ingredients

- 2 tablespoons olive oil, divided
- 1/2 cup diced red onions
- 1 cup sliced mushrooms
- 1/4 cup white wine
- 8 shrimp, peeled and deveined
- 1/2 pound jumbo lump crab meat, picked over but not broken
- 1 tablespoon butter
- 4 (4- to 6-ounce) snapper fillets
- salt and pepper
- 1/4 cup all-purpose flour
- 1/4 cup heavy cream

Direction

- Preheat oven to 500 degrees. In a skillet over medium-high heat, add 1 tablespoon oil. Sauté red onions until translucent. Add mushrooms and cook for 5 minutes. Add wine and cook until almost dry. Add shrimp and cook until just done. Add crab meat and butter and heat until butter is melted.
- Meanwhile, season snapper with salt and pepper, Dredge fish in flour, then cream, then flour again. In a large oven-safe skillet over high heat, sear fish on both sides. Transfer to oven and cook for 4 to 7 minutes (depending on thickness) or until just done. Do not overcook.
- Serve topping over snapper.

298. Sole Fillets In Marsala Cream Recipe

Serving: 4 | Prep: | Cook: 20mins | Ready in:

Ingredients

- 2/3 cup fish stock - See note below
- 8 sole fillets
- 1 Tblsp olive oil
- 1Tbsp butter
- 4 shallots - finely chopped
- 3 1/2 oz baby button mushrooms - cleaned & halved
- 1 Tblsp peppercorns - lightly crushed
- 1/3 cup marsala
- 2/3 pint heavy cream

Direction

- Heat oil & butter in a large skillet.
- Add the shallots & cook for 2 - 3 mins until softened.
- Add the mushrooms & cook for a further 2 - 3 mins until they are just beginning to brown.
- Add the peppercorns & fish to the skillet.
- Fry the fish for 3 - 4 mins on each side or until lightly golden.
- Pour the wine & fish stock over the fish & simmer for 3 mins.
- Carefully remove fish & set aside - keep warm.
- Increase heat & boil mixture in the skillet for about 5 mins or until the sauce has reduced & thickened.
- Stir in the cream.
- Return the fish to the skillet & heat through.
- .
- NOTE:-
- In a pinch, if I didn't have ingredients to make the fish stock, I have used an instant fish/seafood stock mixed with water & had great results.

299. Sole Le Duc Recipe

Serving: 6 | Prep: | Cook: 15mins | Ready in:

Ingredients

- 4 tbsp butter
- 3 Tbsp minced shallots or green onion
- 3/4 tsp.curry powder
- 2 pounds sole fillets, cut crosswise into 1 1/2 wide strips
- 1 Tbsp canned green peppercorns, drained
- 1 Tbsp lemon juice
- 1 cup whipping cream
- salt to taste

Direction

- In wide frying pan over medium heat, melt butter.
- Add shallots, curry, and fish; cook over high heat, shaking pan or pushing fish with a wide spatula to turn(taking care not to break up fish)until fish flakes readily when prodded in thickest portion with a fork(3 to 5 minutes)
- Gently lift fish from pan to serving dish.
- Place peppercorns in a small strainer, rinse with cold water and drain.
- Add to pan with lemon juice and whipping cream.
- Bring to a boil over high heat and cook, stirring, until shiny bubbles form (6 to 8 minutes)
- Drain any juice from fish into pan.
- Return fish to pan, shaking gently to mix with sauce, and heat through.
- Wonderful served with rice and a good... Chablis!

300. Sole With Garlic Lemon And Olives Recipe

Serving: 4 | Prep: | Cook: 20mins | Ready in:

Ingredients

- 4 (1/4 -lb.) sole fillets
- 1/2 cup flour
- 3 Tablespoons olive oil
- 2 large cloves garlic, crushed
- 2 Tablespoons lemon juice
- 10 flavored (marinated) black olives, pitted and chopped
- Pinch crushed red pepper

- 1/4 tsp. salt to taste
- 2 Tablespoons chopped fresh parsley

Direction

- Rinse the fish, then dry them on a paper towels.
- Spread the flour on a plate.
- Warm the oil and garlic in a large skillet.
- Sauté gently till the garlic is golden, then discard it.
- Dust the fish with flour, slip them into the hot oil.
- Sauté until golden, about 1 minute for each filet.
- Transfer to warm plate.
- Reduce heat, stir the lemon juice and 2 tablespoons of water into the pan.
- When the liquid begins to bubble, add the olives, red pepper, salt and parsley.
- Heat briefly, then pour over the fish and serve.

301. Soup With Fish And Pesto Breads Recipe

Serving: 4 | Prep: | Cook: 45mins | Ready in:

Ingredients

- 1 kg milk .
- 2 bay leaves.
- 6 black pepper corns.
- 600 gr fish filet, (cod fish, tilapia or any other firm fish).
- 150 gr Dutch shrimps without shell.
- 2 tbs olive oil.
- 100 gr bacon slices.
- 4 leeks chopped.
- 1 medium onion chopped.
- 2 cloves garlic chopped.
- 2 carots cubed.
- 3 celery stalks chopped.
- 2 potatoes cubed.
- salt and pepper to taste
- 1 ts thyme (dried) if fresh available 2 spriggs.
- 100 gr cream.
- 4 ts parsley chopped.
- shredded peel of 1 lemon.
- 1 tbs lemon juice.
- 1 baquette.
- 4 tbs green pesto.

Direction

- In a big soup pan, warm the milk to medium heat, add dafne and pepper corns and cook for 2 min, add fish and cook another 5 min, take pan from heat and let cool down.
- Heat olive oil in a frying pan to medium heat and sauté the bacon till crispy (8 min), add leeks, carrots, celery, onion, garlic, potatoes and thyme; cook on low heat for 15 min till vegetables are soft.
- Drain the fish and keep the milk, cut fish in chunks and add to vegetables, add milk and simmer for 8 min, add cream, lemon juice, shrimps and cook 4 min more.
- Serve in deep plates, sprinkle with shredded lemon peel and parsley.
- Cut baquette lengthwise in 4 pcs and then each piece in two, put pesto on each side, put in a baking dish and bake 5 min in the preheated oven (180 C), serve with the soup.

302. Southern Fried Catfish Recipe

Serving: 6 | Prep: | Cook: 30mins | Ready in:

Ingredients

- 4-5 lbs catfish fillets
- 1 cup finely ground yellow corn meal
- 1 cup all purpose flour
- 2 tsp salt
- ½-¾ tsp ground black pepper
- 2 tsp granulated garlic
- 2 tsp granulated onion
- ground cayenne pepper to taste

- 2 eggs, beaten
- ½ cup buttermilk
- 1 Tbsp Louisiana style hot sauce
- oil for frying, enough to completely submerge fish

Direction

- Heat oil to 375.
- Rinse catfish fillets and place on paper towel to drain.
- Place corn meal, flour, salt, black and red pepper, granulated garlic and granulated onion in a large shallow bowl and mix well.
- Place eggs, buttermilk, and hot sauce in a bowl and mix well.
- Soak catfish fillets in buttermilk/egg mixture for 5-10 minutes.
- Remove fillets a few at a time from the buttermilk/egg mixture, shake off excess and roll in cornmeal flour mixture.
- Fry in hot oil until golden brown. Season as necessary and serve up hot.
- Note: I use catfish fillets for convenience. The fillets are simple to rinse and cook. If you like, you can use whole catfish. Try to avoid frozen fish. Select smaller fish such as Channel Catfish, dress and skin, leaving tails and fins on. Prepare as noted above.

303. Southern Fried Catfish With 7 Up Recipe

Serving: 4 | Prep: | Cook: 10mins | Ready in:

Ingredients

- catfish fillets (however many you need)
- 1 1/2 teaspoons salt
- 1/4 teaspoon pepper
- 7 oz seven up
- 1 cup yellow cornmeal
- 1/4 cup grits
- oil to fry in

Direction

- Sprinkle fish with salt and pepper.
- Mix cornmeal and grits in separate bowl.
- Dip fish in 7 up then roll in cornmeal mixture.
- Fry fish in hot oil until brown and crisp.
- Drain on paper towel.
- Serve with hushpuppies and tartar sauce.

304. Southwest Catfish Recipe

Serving: 4 | Prep: | Cook: 13mins | Ready in:

Ingredients

- Rub:
- 2 tsp. chili powder
- 2 tsp. granulated garlic
- 2 tsp. paprika
- 2 tsp. kosher / sea salt
- 1 tsp. ground coriander
- 1/2 tsp. cumin
- 1 tsp. ground black pepper
- 4 large catfish filets
- olive oil

Direction

- Combine rub ingredients in small bowl. Gently brush both sides of filets with olive oil. Generously season filets with rub mixture. Rubbing seasoning into fish. Wrap in plastic and refrigerate for 30-45 mins.
- Grill over high heat until the catfish just begins to flake when poked with the tip of a knife, 10-12 mins, turning once. Serve fish warm.

305. Spicy Fried Catfish With Tartar Sauce Recipe

Serving: 6 | Prep: | Cook: 10mins | Ready in:

Ingredients

- 4-6 medium catfish fillets
- 1 1/2 cups plain cornmeal-yellow or white
- 1/2 cup all purpose flour
- 2 teaspoons salt-or to taste
- 1 teaspoon ground black pepper-or to taste
- 1 teaspoon garlic powder-or to taste
- 1 1/2 teaspoons cayenne pepper-or to taste
- 2 cups buttermilk
- 1 tablespoon hot sauce
- oil-peanut,vegetable,corn,or canola
- Tartar Sauce:
- 1 cup mayonaise
- 1/4 cup grated sweet onion
- 1 clove minced fresh garlic or 1 teaspoon granulated garlic
- 1/3 cup chopped sweet pickles
- 1 tablespoon lemon juice
- salt to taste

Direction

- Rinse fillets and pat dry.
- In a shallow dish combine cornmeal, flour, and seasonings. Mix well.
- In a wide medium bowl, combine buttermilk and hot sauce.
- Heat 1/2" to 1" of oil in a large cast iron skillet over medium heat until it reaches 350 degrees.
- Dip each fillet in buttermilk mixture then dredge in cornmeal mixture.
- Fry fish for 5-7 minutes on both sides or until golden brown and flakes easily with fork.
- Drain on paper towels.
- Serve with tartar sauce on the side along with French fries, hushpuppies, and coleslaw.
- Tartar Sauce:
- Mix all ingredients together in a small bowl.
- Cover and refrigerate at least one hour before serving.

306. Spicy Hoisin Salmon Recipe

Serving: 4 | Prep: | Cook: 15mins | Ready in:

Ingredients

- 1/4 c hoisin sauce
- 2Tbs soy sauce
- 2tsp rice vinegar
- 1/2tsp ground ginger
- 1/4tsp red pepper flakes
- 4 pieces salmon filet,about 6 ozs. each
- lemon wedges for garnish

Direction

- Heat oven to 450. Coat a baking dish with cooking spray.
- In a small dish, stir together the hoisin, soy sauce, vinegar, ginger and red pepper flakes. Place salmon in prepared dish and spread top of each filet with hoisin mixture.
- Roast at 450 for 10 mins. Spread remaining hoisin mixture over the salmon and top with the scallions. Roast an additional 5 mins.
- Serve with rice and broccoli and lemon wedges as garnish.

307. Spicy Pickled Salmon Dated 1972 Recipe

Serving: 6 | Prep: | Cook: | Ready in:

Ingredients

- 1 cup water
- 1 cup distilled white vinegar
- 3 tablespoons sugar
- 1/2 teaspoon salt
- 1 small white onion thinly sliced
- 1 lemon thinly sliced
- 1 tablespoon mustard seeds
- 1 teaspoon black peppercorns
- 2 bay leaves

- 3/4 cup firmly packed dill sprigs
- 2 pounds salmon fillet skinned rinsed dried and cut into small pieces

Direction

- Combine water, vinegar, salt, onion, lemon, mustard seeds, peppercorns and bay leaves.
- Bring to a boil over medium high heat stirring until sugar melts.
- Remove from heat and cool.
- Put fish and dill sprigs in glass container and pour cooled vinegar solution over top.
- Stir gently to coat all the pieces then cover and refrigerate at least 24 hours up to 5 days.
- To serve pour off liquid and arrange salmon with the pickled onion and lemon in a bowl.

308. Stout Battered Fish And Chips Recipe

Serving: 6 | Prep: | Cook: 1hours | Ready in:

Ingredients

- 4 Pieces Cod Fillet
- 12 Oz Guinness Stout
- 3/4 Cup Cornstarch
- 3/4 Cup Flour
- 1 3/4 Tbsp Backing Powder
- 1 Tbsp Peanut Oil
- 1/2 Tsp Salt
- Corn Oil or Canola for Fryer
- Salt
- black pepper
- Tarter Sauce
- Lemon Wedges

Direction

- Mix the dry ingredients in a bowl
- .Add the stout a little at a time until you have a nice batter you probably will only need 8 to 10 ounces of the stout. The rest well I drink it.
- Submerge one piece of cod fillet into the batter.
- Meantime your frying oil should be heating up when at 350 degrees F (175 degrees C) it is ready to fry.
- Add the fillet to the oil and submerge the next piece until the frying piece is golden brown. It will be a slightly darker from the color of the stout.
- You should check on the fillet once or twice to make sure it's not sticking.
- When golden brown set on a paper towel and lightly salt and pepper it immediately.
- If you are lucky enough to have a professional deep fryer you can fry more than one at a time.
- Serve with tartar sauce and lemon wedges.
- Don't forget the chips!
- Enjoy and God bless.

309. Strawberry Cajun Cats Recipe

Serving: 4 | Prep: | Cook: 20mins | Ready in:

Ingredients

- 2 pounds catfish fillets
- salt & black pepper
- 2 ounces hot red pepper sauce
- 3/4 cup cornmeal
- 3/4 cup flour
- 2 teaspoons horseradish
- 1 clove garlic, minced
- 1 1/2 cups strawberry preserves
- 1/2 cup safflower oil
- 1/2 cup red wine vinegar
- 1 tablespoon soy sauce
- fresh strawberries
- parsley sprigs, optional
- 1/4 cup seafood cocktail sauce

Direction

- Place fillets in large shallow dish. Season fish with salt, black pepper and hot pepper sauce. Cover and refrigerate 1 hour. In small saucepan, combine preserves, vinegar, soy sauce, cocktail sauce, garlic and horseradish; simmer sauce over low heat stirring occasionally, while preparing catfish. Blend cornmeal and flour in shallow bowl. Heat oil in heavy skillet over medium-high heat. Drain catfish and dredge in cornmeal mixture, coating on all sides. Add catfish to hot pan and sauté until browned on both sides. Drain well on paper towels and keep warm. Spoon 1/4 cup sauce on each plate; top with catfish fillets. Garnish with sliced strawberries and parsley, if desired.
- Note - Strawberry Flavored Vinegar may be used instead of Red Wine Vinegar

310. Stuffed Trout Encassed With Phyllo Recipe

Serving: 4 | Prep: | Cook: 20mins | Ready in:

Ingredients

- 1 filet of whole trout per person
- fresh sliced lemon as needed
- fresh sprigs of rosemary or dill as needed
- 4 sheets of phyllo pastry per fish
- melted butter
- My seafood stuffing:
- some oil or butter to sauté:
- 1 stalk celery fine chopped
- 1 onion chopped
- 1 green bell pepper chopped
- 2 Tbs. fresh chopped parsley
- 1 small carrot coarse grated
- 1 10 oz pkg of baby portabello mushrooms chopped
- 1/2 stick butter melted
- few Tbs. of vermouth or sherry to taste
- 4 to 6 large deli sandwich/ kaiser rolls cubed*
- or day old white bread cubed as needed
- 1 1/2 lbs mixed chopped seafood (shrimp, lobster, crab legs)
- OR use the packaged mock style seafood - which I often use
- Old bay seafood seasoning or favorite fish or seafood seasoning to
- taste

Direction

- Rinse fish well with water and pat dry.
- Salt and pepper fish.
- Set aside.
- Have made prepared seafood stuffing:
- Sauté the vegetable in some butter or olive oil until softened.
- Transfer to a large bowl and add enough bread cubes (amount depends on the size of the rolls) & parsley to make a stuffing.
- Add butter and seasonings to taste.
- Stir in seafood.
- Mix well.
- Stir in some sherry or vermouth.
- Stuffing should be moist but not soggy.
- Stuff insides of fish with desired amount.
- Lay a few lemon slices and a small sprig of rosemary or dill over fish.
- Quickly brush each sheet of phyllo pastry with the butter and wrap/shape the 4 sheets around the fish.
- Brush phyllo enclosed fish with more melted butter.
- Repeat with additional fish.
- Place fish in a well-oiled pan and bake 425F for 20 minutes or until pastry is golden and puffed.
- Serve immediately.
- For a nice appearance plate fish and garnish with lemon wedges & fresh dill or rosemary.
- If desired serve a hollandaise or melted butter on the side if desired.
- Note: the stuffing recipe makes more than needed so bake extra stuffed in a covered casserole for 350F until well heated.
- Also read the package instructions about using phyllo pastry if unfamiliar with its use.

- The pastry sheets are fragile and dry out quickly.

311. Super Simple Salmon Recipe

Serving: 4 | Prep: | Cook: 10mins | Ready in:

Ingredients

- fresh salmon, at least 1/4 lb. per person and 3/4" to 1" thick. (If you are grilling it's better to get salmon with the skin still on)
- Fresh lemon juice, about half a lemon per pound of salmon
- salt or seasoned salt
- dill (fresh or dried)
- Freshly ground pepper
- extra virgin olive oil

Direction

- Rinse the salmon in cold water and pat dry with paper towels.
- Squeeze lemon over one side of fish.
- Drizzle a bit of olive oil over same side.
- Season to your taste with salt, dill and pepper.
- Rub in and repeat on other side.
- Broil or grill 3 to 5 minutes on side one. You will be able to see how done the fish is on the side. Once it's cooked half way through, flip and grill an additional 3 to 5 minutes.
- I serve this with rice and asparagus. Simple, easy and good for you! And the fur kids too!

312. Supreme Salmon Recipe

Serving: 4 | Prep: | Cook: 30mins | Ready in:

Ingredients

- 4 salmon steaks
- salt and pepper
- 2 Tablespoons chopped onions
- 1 Cup cheddar cheese, Shredded
- 1 Cup sour cream
- 1 Tablespoon Chopped parsley
- paprika

Direction

- Place salmon in greased shallow baking dish.
- Sprinkle with salt, pepper and onions.
- Sprinkle with cheese.
- Spoon sour cream over salmon.
- Sprinkle with parsley and paprika.
- Bake 30 minutes in 350 degree oven or until salmon flakes easily.

313. Sushi 101 Recipe

Serving: 2 | Prep: | Cook: 30mins | Ready in:

Ingredients

- 1 bag roasted Seaweed paper (each bag holds 10 sheets)
- 1 1/2 cups white, short-grain rice
- 1/4 cup rice vinegar
- sea salt
- fish of your choice. You can use canned eel like we do, canned albacore, mackrel, even thin cuts of tuna or salmon steak. If you don't 100% trust your local fish market, it's okay to use frozen. Don't take chances with shady products and don't leave fish steaks out while preparing. Be smart!
- Little cup of room temperature water
- Optional: scallions, chopped avacado, spinach chiffonade, eel sauce or spicy mayo.
- Note: If you don't have a special bamboo rolling matt, use either plastic wrap or wax paper. You can even attempt to roll it with your bare hands but it's difficult to get it tight enough that way.

Direction

- Cook white rice well in boiling salted water until soft, use extra water and drain afterwards if you have to.
- Mix drained rice with vinegar.
- On the bamboo rolling matt, place a sheet of roasted seaweed paper, shiny side down.
- Using a spreading knife or a spoon, coat the nearest half of the paper to you with an even coating of rice. It's okay if the rice mixture is a bit liquidy.
- At the very bottom, put a thin line of your fish of choice, and any condiments/additions you want to put with it.
- Using the rolling mechanism, roll up the sushi as tightly as you can going from the bottom up, until you run out of rice. Now only the bare, dry seaweed paper should be showing. With either your fingers or a brush, use a little water you have put aside to moisten top edge of the paper. You may need to be liberal.
- Finish rolling and seal it closed with the moistened end. You know, like a blunt. [=)
- Leave it sitting there with the seam-side down to set for a few minutes before attempting to cut it.
- When you're ready, use a very sharp serrated knife to slice the roll into 6-7 pieces. Serve with premium or sashimi soy sauce.
- Yeah, it really is this easy. Try it!

314. Sweet Bourbon Salmon Recipe

Serving: 4 | Prep: | Cook: 20mins | Ready in:

Ingredients

- 2 8 oz salmon fillets
- 2 tsp chopped chives
- 1 cup bourbon
- 1/4 cup pineapple juice
- 2 Tblsp soy sauce
- 2 Tblsp brown sugar
- 1/4 tsp salt
- 1/4 tsp black pepper
- 1/8 tsp garlic powder
- 1/2 olive oil

Direction

- Combine pineapple juice, brown sugar, bourbon, soy sauce, pepper and garlic powder in a bowl. Stir to dissolve sugar.
- Add the oil.
- Remove any skin on salmon fillets.
- Put fillets in baking dish and pour marinade over and let sit in the fridge for one hour or longer. The longer it can sit, the more the marinade seeps into the fillets.
- Now you can put this on the grill or cook it on the stove top on medium heat. 5-7 minutes per side or until the fillet is cooked to your desire. Brush the marinade over the filets as they are cooking.
- Arrange the fillets on a plate and sprinkle with the chopped chives.
- Service with a brown rice and salad.

315. Sweet N Sour Halibut Recipe

Serving: 2 | Prep: | Cook: 15mins | Ready in:

Ingredients

- 4 to 6 tbsps . sugar
- 1 tbps. cornstarch
- 1/3 cup white vinegar
- 1/4 cup water
- 1 to 2 tps. soy sauce
- 1/4 tps. hot pepper sauce
- 1 tbsp. all-purpose flour
- 1/4 tps. salt
- 1/4 tps. pepper
- 1/2 pound halibut fillet, cut into 2- inch strips
- 2 tbsps. vegetable oil
- 1/2 cup green pepper chunks (1 inch)
- 1/2 cup sweet onion chunks (1 inch)

- 1/2 cup pineapple chunks, drained
- Hot cooked rice

Direction

- 1. In a bowl, combine sugar and cornstarch. Stir in the vinegar, water, soy sauce and hot pepper sauce until smooth; set aside.
- 2. In a small resealable plastic bag combine the flour, salt and pepper. Add fish and shake to coat. In a small skillet, sauté fish in oil for 4-6 minutes or until fish flakes easily with a fork; remove and keep warm
- 3. In same skillet, sauté green pepper and onion for 3 minutes or until crisp-tender. Add pineapple stir sauce and add to skillet. Bring to a boil; cook and stir for 2 minutes or until thickened. Return fish to skillet; heat through. Serve with rice.

316. Sweetly Succulent Mahi Mahi Recipe

Serving: 4 | Prep: | Cook: 12mins | Ready in:

Ingredients

- 3 tablespoons brown sugar
- 4 tbsp water
- 3 tablespoons soy sauce
- 1 tablespoon balsamic vinegar
- 2 teaspoons grated fresh ginger root
- 2 cloves garlic, crushed
- 1 teaspoon olive oil
- 24oz raw mahi mahi fillets, cut in 4
- salt and pepper to taste

Direction

- In a shallow glass dish, stir together the sugar, water, soy sauce, balsamic vinegar, ginger, garlic and olive oil.
- Season fish fillets lightly with salt and pepper, and place them into the dish.
- Cover, and refrigerate for 20 minutes to marinate.
- Preheat broiler.
- Remove fish from the dish, and reserve marinade.
- Place fish on a baking tray and broil 4 to 6 minutes on each side, turning only once, until fish flakes easily with a fork. Remove fillets to a serving platter and keep warm.
- Pour reserved marinade into the skillet, and reduce until the mixture reduces to a glaze.
- Spoon glaze over fish, and serve immediately.

317. Swordfish Sicilian Style Recipe

Serving: 6 | Prep: | Cook: 20mins | Ready in:

Ingredients

- 2Tbs fresh lemon juice
- 2tsp salt
- 2tsp chopped oregano1/4c extra virgin olive oil
- fresh ground pepper
- 2lbs swordfish steaks,cut 1/2" thick.

Direction

- Light a grill. In a small bowl, mix the lemon juice with the salt until the salt dissolves Stir in the oregano. Whisk in the olive oil and season generously with pepper.
- Grill the swordfish steaks over high heat, turning once, until cooked through, 6-7 mins. Transfer the swordfish to a platter. Prick each steak in several places with a fork. Using a spoon, beat the sauce, then drizzle over the fish. Serve at once.

318. Swordfish And Sketti Recipe

Serving: 4 | Prep: | Cook: 20mins | Ready in:

Ingredients

- 1 pound whole-wheat spaghetti
- 1/4 cup water
- 1/2 large onion, peeled and diced
- 1 1/2 pounds peeled ripe tomatoes, diced
- 1 pound kale (preferably Tuscan-style or curly), chopped
- 1 pound swordfish, skinned and cubed into 1/2" pieces
- salt and pepper, to taste
- 1/4 cup arugula, minced

Direction

- In a large pot of boiling, salted water, cook spaghetti until just shy of "al dente" - about 5-6 minutes. Drain and keep warm.
- Heat water in a large skillet.
- Add the onion and sauté 6-7 minutes.
- Add tomatoes and cook 10 minutes.
- Add the kale and swordfish, season to taste, and cook 3 minutes.
- Stir in arugula and cooked spaghetti, tossing well to coat.
- Serve immediately.

319. Swordfish With Tomato Chutney Recipe

Serving: 4 | Prep: | Cook: 8mins | Ready in:

Ingredients

- 2 - 6 to 8 oz. swordfish filets, 3/4 to 1" thick
- chutney
- 1 small leek or 2 green onions, chopped (about 1/4 C)
- 2 tsp olive oil
- 1 C tomato, seeded and chopped
- 1/4 C snipped fresh basi
- 1 Tbl drained capers
- 1/4 tsp ground black pepper
- 1/8 tsp salt
- 2 tsp olive oil

Direction

- Chutney
- In a medium saucepan, cook leek in 2 tsp. hot oil until just tender
- Remove from heat; stir in remaining ingredients and set aside
- Brush 2 tsp. oil over swordfish steaks and grill over medium heat about 6 - 8 minutes per 1/2" thickness, turning once
- Fish should flake easily with a fork
- Serve with chutney

320. TEXAS STYLE COD FILLETS WITH MUSTARD TARRAGON CRUMB CRUST Recipe

Serving: 2 | Prep: | Cook: 20mins | Ready in:

Ingredients

- 4 tablespoons coarse fresh breadcrumbs
- 1 tablespoon chopped fresh tarragon
- 1/2 teaspoon grated lemon zest
- 2 teaspoons melted butter
- 1 teaspoon salt
- 2 teaspoons freshly ground black pepper
- 2 cod fillets
- 1/2 teaspoon Dijon mustard

Direction

- Heat the oven to 450.
- In a small bowl gently mix breadcrumbs, tarragon, lemon zest, melted butter, salt and pepper.
- Spread each fillet with 1/4 teaspoon mustard.

- Carefully pat the crumb topping over the surface of each fillet pressing lightly so it sticks.
- Brush a little oil onto a small baking sheet or shallow baking pan and set the fillets on the oiled spot.
- Bake fish in the hot oven until the topping is golden brown and crisp and the fish is tender all the way through when you poke it with a thin knife or a skewer 10 to 15 minutes.
- Serve immediately.

321. Talapia With Cucumber Radish Relish Recipe

Serving: 4 | Prep: | Cook: 5mins | Ready in:

Ingredients

- 2/3 cup chopped, seeded cucumber
- 1/2 cup chopped radishes
- 1 teaspoon vegetable oil
- 2 tablespoons tarragon vinegar
- 1/4 teaspoon dried tarragon
- pinch of sugar
- 1/8 teaspoon salt
- 4 (6 oz.) tilapia fillets
- 2 tablespoons margarine

Direction

- Combine the first seven ingredients in a small bowl; mix well.
- Let stand at room temperature while preparing fish.
- Sauté tilapia in margarine in a large skillet over medium heat for 2 to 3 minutes on each side or until fish just begins to flake easily when tested with a fork.
- Transfer to serving plates.
- Spoon cucumber mixture over each serving.

322. Tasty Salmon Filet Recipe

Serving: 2 | Prep: | Cook: 20mins | Ready in:

Ingredients

- 1 salmon fillet (half a salmon, skin on)
- dried tarragon
- dill weed
- granulated garlic (or powder)
- smoked paprika
- dried basil
- lemon peel
- salt
- butter (not necessary, but I did anyway)
- pepper

Direction

- This is what I do: Double some aluminum foil about 2 feet long
- Put on cookie sheet or other baking pan
- Place salmon skin side down on foil
- Sprinkle and rub all ingredients in equal portions on salmon (you choose amount)
- Dot with butter on top
- Seal foil around salmon pinching it closed, trying to keep above salmon, not touching it, just creating a tent so to speak
- Bake (or grill) in 375*F oven for approx. 20 min. depending on thickness of salmon (mine was perfect in 21 min - about 1" thick at biggest part) Do not overcook - it continues to cook a while when taken out of oven - if anything take out when you think it is almost done. It's better underdone than overdone.
- Usually comes off skin when lifted carefully with metal spatula or just scrape off on plate.

323. Tasty Salmon Pie With Dill Sauce Recipe

Serving: 6 | Prep: | Cook: 50mins | Ready in:

Ingredients

- Crust Ingredients:
- 1/4 cup butter
- 3/4 cup finely crushed dried crumbly-style herb seasoned stuffing
- ==========
- Filling Ingredients:
- 2 cups crushed dried crumbly-style herb seasoned stuffing
- 4 ounces (1 cup) cheddar cheese, shredded
- 1 cup water
- 1/2 cup milk
- 1 (16-ounce) can red salmon, drained, skin and bones removed, flaked*
- 2 eggs
- 2 tablespoons chopped fresh parsley
- 1 tablespoon finely chopped onion
- 1 teaspoon instant chicken bouillon granules
- 1/2 teaspoon dry mustard
- ==========
- Sauce Ingredients:
- 1/3 cup butter
- 2 tablespoons cornstarch
- 1 1/3 cups water
- 1 teaspoon dried dill weed
- 1/2 teaspoon salt
- 2 medium (2 cups) tomatoes, cubed 1/2-inch

Direction

- Heat oven to 350°F. Melt 1/4 cup butter in 3-quart saucepan; stir in 3/4 cup finely crushed stuffing. Press stuffing mixture on bottom and up sides of greased 9-inch pie pan; set aside.
- Stir together all filling ingredients in same saucepan; spoon into crust. Bake for 50 to 55 minutes or until heated through. Let stand 10 minutes.
- Meanwhile, melt 1/3 cup butter in 2-quart saucepan. Stir in cornstarch. Stir in all remaining sauce ingredients except tomatoes. Cook over medium heat, stirring occasionally, until mixture comes to a full boil (5 to 7 minutes). Add tomatoes; boil 1 minute.
- To serve, cut pie into 6 wedges; serve sauce over wedges.
- *Substitute 3 (6 1/8-ounce) cans tuna, drained, and flaked.

324. Teriyaki Grilled Salmon Recipe

Serving: 4 | Prep: | Cook: 12mins | Ready in:

Ingredients

- 3 tablespoons oil
- 3 tablespoons soy sauce
- 1 1/2 tablespoons minced fresh garlic
- 1 1/2 tablespoons minced fresh ginger
- 4 4-ounce Alaska salmon steaks or fillets (4 to 6 ounces each)
- 1 sheet (12 × 18 inch) Reynolds wrap heavy duty aluminum foil

Direction

- In a shallow baking dish, combine brown sugar, oil, soy sauce, garlic and ginger.
- Place Alaska salmon steaks/fillets in a baking dish. Turn fish over several times to coat; refrigerate 30 to 45 minutes.
- Remove salmon from marinade.
- Cook on foil sheet on medium hot grill, turning once during cooking, about 6 to 12 minutes per inch of thickness.
- Do not overcook.
- ENJOY.....

325. Teriyaki Salmon

Serving: 0 | Prep: | Cook: | Ready in:

Ingredients

- ¼ cup sesame oil
- ¼ cup lemon juice
- ¼ cup soy sauce
- 2 tablespoons brown sugar, or more to taste

- 1 tablespoon sesame seeds
- 1 teaspoon ground mustard
- 1 teaspoon ground ginger
- ¼ teaspoon garlic powder
- 4 (6 ounce) salmon steaks

Direction

- Mix sesame oil, lemon juice, soy sauce, brown sugar, sesame seeds, ground mustard, ginger, and garlic powder in a small saucepan over low heat. Bring to a simmer, stirring until sugar has dissolved. Set aside 1/2 cup of marinade for basting.
- Pour remaining marinade into a resealable plastic bag and place salmon into the marinade. Squeeze air out of the bag, seal, and marinate the salmon steaks for at least 1 hour (2 hours for better flavor). Drain and discard used marinade.
- Set oven rack about 4 inches from the heat source and preheat the oven's broiler. Place salmon steaks into a broiler pan and broil for 5 minutes. Brush steaks with reserved marinade, turn, and broil until fish is opaque and flakes easily, about 5 more minutes. Brush again with marinade.
- Nutrition Facts
- Per Serving:
- 410.8 calories; protein 33.6g 67% DV; carbohydrates 10.3g 3% DV; fat 25.8g 40% DV; cholesterol 82.5mg 28% DV; sodium 972.6mg 39% DV.

326. Teriyaki Salmon Recipe

Serving: 4 | Prep: | Cook: 10mins | Ready in:

Ingredients

- 4 salmon steaks skinned
- 1 1/4 cup soy sauce
- 1/3 cup sake
- 6 tablespoons granulated sugar
- 3 garlic cloves minced
- 1 tablespoon minced ginger root
- 1/3 cup vegetable oil

Direction

- Combine all ingredients for the marinade in a small bowl and stir until sugar dissolves.
- To prepare salmon quickly rinse under cold running water and pat dry with paper towels.
- Divide each steak into 2 pieces by cutting along either side of the central bone.
- Discard bone the cut fillet into 8 equal pieces.
- Place salmon in a shallow glass or ceramic container and pour 1 cup marinade over the fish.
- Cover and refrigerate for 2 hours turning fish occasionally.
- Let come to room temperature before cooking.
- Remove salmon from marinade reserving the marinade.
- Place fish on an oiled grill rack.
- Position fish 6 inches from heat source turning once.
- Bush several times with the reserved marinade and cook 5 minutes per side.
- Serve salmon immediately with reserved marinade as dipping sauce.

327. Teriyaki Salmon And Green Onion Kabobs Recipe

Serving: 6 | Prep: | Cook: 10mins | Ready in:

Ingredients

- 3/4 cup teriyaki marinade
- 3 tablespoons minced fresh ginger
- 2 tablespoons minced garlic
- 1 tablespoon sugar
- 1/8 teaspoon hot chili flakes
- 2 pounds boned skinned salmon fillet rinsed patted dry and cut into cubes
- vegetable oil for grill
- 2 bunches green onions cut into 1" lengths

Direction

- In a medium bowl mix marinade, ginger, garlic, sugar and chili flakes. Add salmon and mix gently to coat. Cover and refrigerate 45 minutes. Prepare a gas grill for direct high heat. When hot brush grill with a generous coat of oil. While grill heats thread cubes of fish onto skewers alternating with pieces of green onion. Lay skewers on grill and cook about 4 minutes. Using two spatulas gently turn each skewer over and cook 4 minutes on other side.

328. Tex Mex Salmon Recipe

Serving: 4 | Prep: | Cook: 11mins | Ready in:

Ingredients

- 4 6-oz. salmon steaks
- 2 fresh jalapeno Chiles, seeded, and finely chopped
- 2 Tbsp capers, drained
- 1/3 cup thinly-sliced pimento-stuffed green olives
- 3 Tbsp finely chopped fresh cilantro
- 2 Tbsp olive oil
- 1 large onion, chopped
- 2 cloves garlic, minced
- 4 tsp sugar
- 1 tsp salt
- 1/4 tsp ground cinnamon
- 1/4 tsp ground cloves
- 4 cups tomato puree
- 1 1/2 tsp lemon juice
- 1 1/2 tsp water
- 1 Tbsp cornstarch

Direction

- Heat the oil in a wide frying pan over medium heat.
- Add the onion and garlic and cook, stirring often, until the onion is soft. Stir in the sugar, salt, cinnamon, cloves, and puree.
- Cook over high heat until a thick sauce forms.
- Blend the lemon juice, water and cornstarch together, and stir into the tomato mixture.
- Cook until the mixture boils.
- Nestle the salmon steaks into the sauce, cover and cook over medium-high heat for about 4 minutes. Then turn the salmon steaks, cover and cook another 4-5 minutes, or until the salmon begins to flake at the touch of a fork.
- Add the chilies and capers, and cook another 2-3 minutes.
- To serve, place the steaks on individual plates, and surround and top the fish with the sauce.

329. Thai Style Tilapia Recipe

Serving: 45 | Prep: | Cook: 15mins | Ready in:

Ingredients

- 1 cup coconut milk
- 6 whole almonds
- 2 Tbs chopped white onion
- 1 tsp ground ginger
- 1/2 tsp ground turmeric
- 1 tsp chopped fresh lemon grass (I never have this)
- 1/4 tsp salt
- 4 or 5 fillets tilapia
- salt and pepper to tast
- 1/2 tsp red pepper flakes or to taste

Direction

- 1. In a food processor or blender, combine the coconut milk, almonds, onion, ginger, turmeric, lemon grass, and 1/4 tsp. salt process till smooth
- 2. Heat a large non-stick skillet over medium-high heat. Season the fish fillets with salt and pepper on both sides then place them skin-side up in the skillet. Pour the pureed sauce

over the fish. Use a spatula to coat the fish evenly with the sauce. Sprinkle with red pepper flakes.

- 3. Reduce heat to medium, cover, and simmer for about 15 minutes, until the puree is thickened and fish flakes easily with a fork.

330. Thai Styled Basa With Almond Crust And Sweet Chili Glaze Recipe

Serving: 4 | Prep: | Cook: 12mins | Ready in:

Ingredients

- 4 basa fillets, about ½ lb each (you could use flounder, catfish or any thick white fish)
- 1/3 c. ground almond
- 1 small bunch fresh basil leaves, chopped finely
- 2 t. cajun seasoning
- 2 T. cream sherry
- 2 T. nut oil, walnut, almond or peanut
- 1-2 t. hot sauce, optional
- 4 T. Thai sweet chili sauce
- olive oil spray

Direction

- Preheat oven to 450 degrees.
- Combine almond, basil, Cajun seasoning, sherry and oil. Test for spiciness and add hot sauce as desired.
- Spray a baking pan thoroughly with olive oil spray. Place fish filet in pan and cover with the almond paste. Pat down. Spray with a bit more olive oil spray.
- Cook until the fish is done and the crust gets "crusty". Spoon chili sauce on each filet. Cook about 2 minutes more until sauce begins to glaze.

331. The Baked Flounder Recipe

Serving: 4 | Prep: | Cook: 18mins | Ready in:

Ingredients

- * 2 lemons, sliced into 1/4-inch-thick rounds
- * 2 medium onions, sliced into very thin rounds (8 ounces ea.)
- * 4 tablespoons unsalted butter
- * 1 cup dry white wine
- * 1 teaspoon chopped fresh thyme, plus 4 sprigs
- * coarse salt and freshly ground pepper
- * 4 six-ounce flounder fillets (or other white fish)

Direction

- Preheat oven to 400°.
- Arrange lemons and onions in a 9-by-13-inch glass baking dish.
- Dot with butter; add wine and 1/4 cup cold water.
- Sprinkle with chopped thyme; season with salt and pepper.
- Bake until onions are soft and translucent, about 40 minutes.
- Remove baking dish from oven.
- Arrange fish fillets over lemons and onions.
- Season fillets with salt and pepper.
- Scatter thyme sprigs over fish.
- Baste fish with a little cooking liquid.
- Bake until fish is just opaque and cooked through 16 to 18 minutes.
- Do not overcook.
- Serve fish with cooked onions and lemons.

332. Tilapia Biryani Recipe

Serving: 6 | Prep: | Cook: 60mins | Ready in:

Ingredients

- 5 tilapia fish filets
- 2 tbs butter
- 4 cloves garlic, peeled and chopped
- 1 thumb-size length of ginger, peeled and chopped
- 1 tsp chilli powder
- 1 tsp turmeric powder
- 1 tspp cumin powder
- 1 tsp sea salt
- masala vegetables
- 2 tbs butter
- 2 tbs garam masala
- a handful of raw cashews
- 1 red onion, peeled and sliced into thin rounds
- 3 serrano green chilies chopped
- 1 thumb-size length of ginger, peeled and chopped
- 4 cloves garlic, peeled and chopped
- 1 tomato diced
- 1/2 cup green peas
- 4 leaves of kale sliced into strips
- 3 small purple potatoes
- rice
- 3 cups basmati rice
- 1 tbs butter
- 2 cloves garlic, smashed
- 1 red onion, peeled and chopped
- 5 cm stick cinnamon
- 2 cardamom pods the green ones
- 5 -6 cloves
- 1 tsp saffron threads
- 1 tsp sea salt
- 3 cups unsalted stock or water
- 1/2 cup of equal parts chopped mint and cilantro
- Garnish
- 4 tbs yogurt
- Fried red onions
- fresh cilantro leaves

Direction

- Fish: Heat oil in a wok and brown the chopped onion, garlic and ginger. Add a little water to the spice powders to make a paste and fry over a moderate fire till fragrant.
- Add salt. Turn the fish until firm and browned and remove from the wok save any leftover oil to flavor the rice. Set fish aside.
- Rice: Wash and drain the rice. In a rice cooker, add the reserved butter and rice grains. Pour stock over the rice. Add salt, saffron threads and 1/2 cup of equal parts chopped mint and cilantro stir to evenly distribute spices etc.
- Set rice cooker program for white rice and cook till the cooker beeps.
- While the rice is cooking, combine and stir fry the masala vegetable ingredients until they are toasted and the spices are evenly distributed.
- When the rice is done, fluff the rice and get an oven-safe pot.
- Layer the rice then the fish then rice then the veggies, then the rice until everything is in the pot.
- Bake for 30-40 minutes at 350.
- Remove the layers into separate serving dishes i.e. rice, fish, veggies.
- Serve with fried red onions and yogurt on the side.

333. Tilapia Fajitas Recipe

Serving: 5 | Prep: | Cook: 20mins | Ready in:

Ingredients

- 1-1/2 Pounds - tilapia fillets
- 1/8 Teaspoon - garlic powder
- 1/8 Teaspoon - chili powder
- 1/8 Teaspoon - fresh ground black pepper
- 1 Tablespoon - lime juice
- 1/4 Teaspoon - Crushed Red hot pepper
- 2 Teaspoons - worcestershire sauce
- 2 Tablespoons - vegetable oil (I use extra virgin olive oil.......)
- 1 - onion (Thinly sliced)
- 1 - green bell pepper (Thinly Sliced)
- 1 - red bell pepper (Thinly Sliced)
- 1 - tomato (Diced) Optional
- salt to Taste

- fresh ground black pepper to Taste
- 10 - 10-inch flour tortillas
- Toppings:
- chunky salsa
- guacamole
- cheddar cheese
- sour cream

Direction

- Combine garlic powder, chili powder, pepper, lime juice, crushed red pepper and Worcestershire sauce in a bowl. Transfer to a shallow pan or large ziplock bag. (I use the baggie!!)
- Place tilapia in pan or baggie and marinate fillets 30 minutes to 1 hour.
- Heat oil in large frying pan on medium heat.
- Sauté onions, for 5 minutes, add peppers and cook until just hot; season to taste with salt and pepper.
- Place peppers and onions on a serving dish.
- Keep hot.
- Remove tilapia fillets from marinade and cook in frying pan on medium heat until fish flakes easily with fork.
- Place finished fish on serving dish over peppers and onions.
- Serve with tortillas, salsa (or diced tomatoes), guacamole, shredded cheese and sour cream.
- Note: The diced tomato can be used in place of the salsa or lightly cooked with the onions and bell pepper.
- Note: Steamed corn tortillas can be used in place of the flour tortillas.
- Enjoy!!!

334. Tilapia Florentine Recipe

Serving: 4 | Prep: | Cook: 30mins | Ready in:

Ingredients

- 1 pkg (6oz) baby spinach
- 6 tsp. canola oil,divided
- 4 tilapia fillets(4oz ea)
- 2Tbs lime juice
- 2tsp garlic-herb seasoning blend
- 1 egg ,lightly beaten
- 1/2c part-skim ricotta cheese
- 1/4c grated parmesan cheese

Direction

- In a non-stick skillet, cook spinach in 4 tsp oil till wilted; drain.
- Meanwhile, place tilapia fillets in greased 9x13" baking dish. Drizzle with lime juice and remaining oil. Sprinkle with seasoning blend.
- In a small bowl, combine the egg, ricotta cheese and spinach; spoon over fillets. Sprinkle with parmesan cheese.
- Bake at 375 for 15-20 mins or till fish flakes easily with a fork.

335. Tilapia Parmesan Saut Recipe

Serving: 4 | Prep: | Cook: 6mins | Ready in:

Ingredients

- 4 6 Rain Forest tilapia fillets
- 1 Tablespoon olive oil
- 1/4 cup grated parmesan cheese
- 2 Tablespoons parsley flakes
- 2 Tablespoons butter
- 1 Tablespoon lemon juice
- 1 Teaspoon garlic powder

Direction

- Mix Parmesan cheese, garlic powder, parsley flakes; set aside.
- Heat a large sauté pan and add olive oil, butter, and lemon.
- Sauté fillets 2-3 minutes per side until white and flaky.
- Sprinkle cheese mixture on fillets and sauté each side for another minute, then serve.

336. Tilapia With Green Curry Recipe

Serving: 4 | Prep: | Cook: 20mins | Ready in:

Ingredients

- About 1 1/2 pounds tilapia or other fish fillets
- 1/4 cup coconut oil or vegetable oil
- 2 teaspoons black mustard seeds
- 1/2 cup fresh or frozen curry leaves
- 2 cups water (1 cup if using tomato)
- 4 to 6 pieces fish tamarind, or substitute 1 cup chopped (preferably green) tomatoes
- 1 1/4 teaspoon salt
- masala Paste:
- 3 tablespoons chopped ginger
- 1 tablespoon chopped garlic
- 1/2 cup chopped shallots
- 6 green cayenne chiles, seeded and coarsely chopped
- 1/2 cup packed coriander leaves and stems
- 1/2 cup fresh or frozen grated coconut, or substitute dried shredded coconut:coconut mixed with 1 tablespoon water
- 1 teaspoon ground coriander
- 1 teaspoon turmeric
- Tempering:
- About 4 tablespoons ghee or butter
- 4 to 6 fresh or frozen curry leaves
- 1/2 cup sliced shallots
- 2 tablespoons minced garlic* or *garlic mashed to a paste
- 3 green cayenne chiles, stemmed and cut in half

Direction

- Rinse the fish fillets, cut into 2-inch pieces, and set aside.
- To prepare the masala paste, place the ginger, garlic, shallots, chiles, and fresh coriander in a food processor, mini-chopper, or stone mortar and process or grind to a coarse paste. Add the coconut and process or grind to a paste (if the mixture seems dry, add a little water as necessary to make a paste). Transfer to a bowl and stir in the ground coriander and turmeric; set aside.
- To prepare the tempering, heat the ghee or butter in a medium heavy skillet over medium-high heat. Toss in the curry leaves, wait a moment, then add the shallots and garlic. Lower the heat to medium and cook until starting to soften, for about 4 minutes, stirring occasionally. Add the chiles and cook until the shallots are very soft and touched with brown, about 5 minutes more. Set aside.
- Heat the oil in a wok or karahi or a heavy pot over medium-high heat. Add the mustard seeds, and when they have popped, add the curry leaves and masala paste. Lower the heat to medium and cook, stirring occasionally, until the oil rises to the surface, about 5 minutes. Add the water and fish tamarind or tomatoes and bring to a boil. Add the salt and the fish and simmer, turning the fish once, for 3 to 5 minutes, until just barely cooked through.
- Add the tempering mixture and simmer for a minute, then serve hot.

337. Tilapia With Mango Salsa Recipe

Serving: 2 | Prep: | Cook: 6mins | Ready in:

Ingredients

- 2 tsp reduced-calorie balsamic vinegar
- 1 mango
- 1 tsp chopped jalapeno pepper
- 1/4 cup finely chopped cucumber
- 2 tsp grated lime zest
- 2 tbsp finely chopped red onion
- 2 tilapia fillets (about 1/2 lb)
- 2 tsp canola oil

- 1/2 cup uncooked brown rice
- salt & pepper to taste

Direction

- Slice mango close to the pit
- Make diagonal cuts through the fruit, leaving the skin intact
- Now invert the peel, and gently pare off the little cubes of fruit
- Finely chop the cucumber, jalapeno and onion
- Combine all ingredients as chopped
- Add the balsamic vinegar
- ===========
- Meanwhile, cook the rice and drain
- ===========
- Cook the tilapia over medium-high flame for three minutes per side, (I cook with propane gas) in a small amount of canola oil and balsamic vinegar
- ===========
- To plate:
- Place a bed of rice in the center of the dish
- Place tilapia on top
- Cover with salsa, OR place a dab of salsa on the fish, and surround the bed of rice with salsa to compliment

338. Tilapia With Tomatoes And Olives Recipe

Serving: 6 | Prep: | Cook: 20mins | Ready in:

Ingredients

- 6 tilapia fillets
- 1/4 cup EVOO
- 4 sprigs of fresh thyme
- 3 TBL. chopped fresh parsley
- 3 tomatoes, peeled, seeded and chopped
- 1/2 cup coarsely chopped green olives
- 1/4 tsp. dried hot red pepper flakes
- 2 garlic cloves, minced
- 1/2 cup finely chopped red onion (I used 2 green onions chopped)
- 1 Tbl. fresh lime juice

Direction

- Preheat oven to 400 degrees
- Lightly oil a shallow baking dish large enough to hold the fillets in one layer.
- In a bowl, stir together the oil, thyme, parsley, tomatoes, olives, onion, red pepper flakes, garlic and lime juice.
- In the prepared baking dish arrange fillets, skin sides down, season them with salt and pepper and spoon the tomato mixture over them.
- Bake the fish, uncovered, in the middle of the oven for 15 to 20 minutes or until it just flakes.

339. Tinks Chateau Libido Fettuccine In Salmon Basil Sauce Recipe

Serving: 4 | Prep: | Cook: 15mins | Ready in:

Ingredients

- 2-- Tablespoon butter........................
- 8- ounces fresh salmon, boned and cut into 3/4" dice or you can use smoked salmon cut in to ribbon strips ....
- 1 -small onion, minced ....
- 1 - tomato, chopped ....
- 1/4- cup Sauternes or other dry white wine......................
- 1 3/4 lb-. fettuccine........................
- 1- 2 -Tablespoon butter........................
- 1/2 cup whipping cream ....
- 3 Tablespoon finely chopped fresh basil ....
- 1 -Tablespoon minced fresh parsley...........
- salt and freshly ground pepper to taste ....
- extra butter for sauteeing salmon

Direction

- Cook fettuccine according to package directions until al dente. Drain and move to warmed pasta bowl.
- Toss with butter.
- Sauté fresh salmon in a skillet with more butter or olive oil remove or if using smoked no need to heat unless you want to.
- Add cream and basil -wine and 1-2-tablespoons butter to frying pan.
- Bring heat to high and boil until sauce thickens slightly.
- Turn heat to low.
- Gently fold in sautéed salmon or smoked salmon, parsley, pepper, and salt.
- Pour sauce over pasta and toss gently; toss onions and tomatoes on top.
- Serve with crusty French bread and a bottle of your favorite wine

340. Tonys Fried Sea Bass With Leeks And Creamy Coconut Grits Recipe

Serving: 4 | Prep: | Cook: 15mins | Ready in:

Ingredients

- For Fried Fish:
- 4 Chilean sea bass fillets (center cut, no skin)
- 2 cups Sweet rice flour
- 1 tbsp white pepper
- 1 tbsp kosher salt
- chili oil(to taste)
- canola oil for frying
- ~~~~~~
- Sauce:
- 1 large leek, cleaned and thinly sliced (white & light green part only)
- 7 garlic cloves, peeled and minced
- 2 tbsp fish sauce
- 1Tbsp lime juice
- ½ cup sugar
- water
- ~~~~~~
- coconut Grits:
- 4 fresh shitake mushrooms, fine dice
- Quick grits (4 servings worth)
- ½ cup coconut milk
- ~~~~~~
- Garnish:
- Saifun noodle threads, fried
- nori (dried sea weed sheet), julienned

Direction

- Season sea bass fillets with white pepper and salt, dredge in rice flour.
- In a non-stick skillet, bring canola oil and chili oil up to temp for shallow frying. After flipping the fillets, spoon oil over the fillets while frying the other side. Pan-fry fillets for approx. 4 mins per side depending on thickness. Using a thermometer, the center should be 130 degrees.
- For the sauce, sprinkle garlic with salt. Strain the garlic and salt in a sauce pan thru a strainer using about 3 cups warm water. Discard minced garlic. Add sugar, fish sauce, and lime juice. Bring to a boil, reduce heat to medium and cook for 20 mins so sauce will thicken slightly (sauce should be delicate, and not too thick). Add leeks to the sauce and cook for about the last 10 minutes until tender.
- In a small pot, add water and bring to boil, add quick grits, and shitake mushrooms, stirring occasionally. Once grits start to thicken after 4 minutes, add coconut milk (cream) stir for about a minute or two more. The grits will thicken up more after removed from heat.
- In a shallow serving bowl, add a dollop of coconut grits, put fish on top, spoon some of the leeks on top of the fish, ladle some of the sauce around the bowl, garnish with saifun noodle and nori.

341. Traditional Style Kedgeree Recipe

Serving: 4 | Prep: | Cook: 2hours | Ready in:

Ingredients

- 450g/1lb Smoked Haddock fillets - all bones removed
- 60g/2oz Ghee or butter
- 1 clove Garlic - finely chopped
- 180g/6oz basmati rice
- 1½in/4cm fresh Ginger - grated
- 4tbsp Spring Onions - finely chopped
- 2tbsp medium Curry Powder
- 2 Tomatoes - peeled, deseeded and chopped
- 1tsp Dijon Mustard
- Handful fresh Coriander - torn and shredded
- 150ml?5fl oz chicken stock
- 1 Bay Leaf
- ½ Lemon - juice only - to taste
- 1 small fresh Red Chilli - seeds removed - finely chopped
- 2 large Eggs - hard boiled
- Salt and freshly ground black pepper

Direction

- Cook the rice, drain, cool and set aside.
- Boil the eggs for some 10 minutes or so, drain, cool and set aside.
- Place the fish and bay leaves and a little salt in a shallow pan and cover with milk/water or mixture of both.
- Bring to the boil, cover and, reducing heat, simmer for about 5 minutes or so or until fish just cooked through.
- Remove from pan and leave to cool.
- Remove the skin from fish, flake into chunks and set aside.
- Melt the butter in a pan over a low heat, add the ginger, onion and garlic and cook for some 5 minutes or so to soften.
- Add the curry powder and mustard, stir in well and cook for a further few minutes.
- Add the chopped tomatoes, chicken stock and lemon juice; stir in well and, increasing heat, bring to a boil.
- Reduce heat to gentle, add the fish and rice to the pan and, stirring gently, heat through.
- Shell and Quarter the eggs.
- Add the eggs, most of the coriander and the chili and stir gently to consistency desired.
- Serve on plates adding the rest of the coriander as garnish.

342. Trout With Tomato Cilantro Linguine Recipe

Serving: 4 | Prep: | Cook: 20mins | Ready in:

Ingredients

- 2 tablespoons olive oil
- 1-1/2 tablespoons fresh lime juice
- 1 tablespoon drained capers
- 4 small roma tomatoes seeded and chopped
- 2 garlic cloves minced
- 1/4 teaspoon cayenne pepper
- 1/3 cup fresh cilantro leaves
- 4 trout steaks
- 1/4 teaspoon salt
- 1 teaspoon freshly ground black pepper
- olive oil or cooking spray
- 10 ounces fresh linguine

Direction

- Stir together oil, juice, capers, tomatoes, garlic, red pepper and cilantro then set aside.
- Remove and discard any skin from fish then rinse and pat dry.
- Cut fish into 4 serving pieces then season with salt and black pepper.
- Spray wide nonstick frying pan with cooking spray and place over medium high heat.
- Add fish and cook 8 minutes turning once.
- Meanwhile in 6 quart pan cook linguine in boiling water for 2 minutes then drain well.

- Set 2 tablespoons tomato mixture aside then lightly mix remaining mix with hot pasta.
- Divide pasta among 4 warm plates and top each serving with a piece of fish.
- Top fish evenly with reserved tomato mixture.

343. Trout Stuff With Fresh Mint And Basil Recipe

Serving: 2 | Prep: | Cook: 18mins | Ready in:

Ingredients

- one filet of trout
- fresh mint
- fresh basil
- sea salt
- olive oil

Direction

- Turn oven on to 375.
- Clean the filet of trout and dry.
- Cut in big piece the mint and the basil.
- Cut filet in half.
- Put the herb on one of the filet.
- Salt to taste.
- Put the other filet on the top.
- Put in oven-ready pan.
- Cook in oven for 18 mins.

344. Tuna And White Bean Salad Recipe

Serving: 6 | Prep: | Cook: 8mins | Ready in:

Ingredients

- 2 15 ounce cans cannellini or great northern beans, rinsed and drained
- 3 Large roma tomatoes, seeded and chopped (about 1 1/2 cups)
- 1/2 C chopped fennel, reserve leafy tops
- 1/3 C chopped red onion
- 1/3 C orange or red bell pepper
- 1 Tbl snipped fennel leaf tops
- 1/4 c EVOO
- 3 Tbl white wine vinegar
- 2 Tbl lemon juice
- 1/4 tsp salt
- 1/4 tsp pepper
- 1 6 ounce tuna steak, cut 1 inch thick
- or
- 2 3 ounce pouches of albacore tuna
- salt
- ground black pepper
- 1 Tbl EVOO
- 2 C torn mixed salad greens
- Leafy fennel tops

Direction

- Salad:
- In a large bowl, combine beans, tomatoes, chopped fennel, red onion, sweet pepper and the snipped fennel tops; set aside.
- Vinaigrette:
- In a screw top jar, combine the 1/4 c oil, the vinegar, lemon juice, 1/4 tsp each of salt and pepper.
- Cover and shake well.
- Pour dressing over bean mixture; gently toss to coat.
- Let stand at room temperature 30 minutes.
- Sprinkle tuna, if using fresh, with salt and pepper; heat 1 tbsp oil over medium high.
- Add tuna and cook for 8 to 12 minutes or until fish flakes easily with a fork, turning once.
- Break tuna into pieces.
- Add tuna to bean mixture; toss to combine.
- Line a serving platter with salad greens, spoon bean mixture over greens.
- Garnish with additional fennel tops, if desired.

345. Tuna Tartare With Olive Crustini Recipe

Serving: 8 | Prep: | Cook: 5mins | Ready in:

Ingredients

- 1 ¼ lb sushi grade tuna fillet, finely chopped
- ¼ cup plus 2 Tablespoons extra-virgin olive oil
- Mixed green, whit, pink, and black peppercorn
- ½ cup finely chopped fennel bulb plus fronds for garnish
- ¼ cup fresh lemon juice
- Coarse salt
- 4 slices of coarse country bread, 4inches square and ½ inch thick, crust removed
- OLIVE SPREAD
- 1 Tablespoon pine nuts
- ¾ cup brine-cured green olives, pitted
- 2 Tablespoons chopped red onion
- 2 cloves garlic, chopped
- 1 Tablespoon olive oil

Direction

- In a medium bowl combine tuna, ¼ cup olive oil and the ground peppercorn to taste, mixing well. If desired cover and refrigerate for at least 30 minutes or up to 3 hours to chill.
- To make olive spread toast the pine nuts in small frying pan over medium heat, stirring constantly, until golden, about 4 minutes. Pour onto plate to cool. In a blender or food processor combine the nuts, olives, red onion, garlic, and olive oil and process until smooth. Set aside.
- Preheat the broiler. Arrange the bread on a baking sheet and toast, turning once, until crisp about 5 minutes in total. Let cool and cut into 16 strips about 1 inch thick.
- Brush strips with olive oil and spread with the olive spread.
- In a small bowl mix together the chopped fennel, lemon juice, and 1 teaspoon of salt.
- Just before serving add the fennel mixture to the chilled season tuna mixing well. Taste and adjust the seasoning. Garnish with fennel fronds. Serve with toasts.
- Optional can add a spoonful of Dijon Mustard to the Tuna Tartar Mix

346. Tuna Tartare With Wasabi Recipe

Serving: 4 | Prep: | Cook: | Ready in:

Ingredients

- 1 pound very fresh tuna steak
- 1/2 cup grape seed oil
- juice and zest of 2 limes
- 1/2 cup freshly squeezed lime juice
- 1 1/2 teaspoons wasabi powder
- 1 tablespoon soy sauce
- 1/2 teaspoon Tabasco sauce
- 1 tablespoons salt
- 1 1/2 teaspoons freshly ground black pepper
- 1/2cups minced scallions, white and green parts (12 scallions)
- 2 avocados
- Extremely finely julienned vegetables: preferably Asian vegetables, but also cucumbers, carrots, celery, -- whatever is lovely, crisp, and extraordinarily fresh
- 1 1/2 tablespoons toasted sesame seeds

Direction

- Combine the oil, lime zest, lime juice, wasabi, soy sauce, Tabasco, salt, and pepper in a bowl. Cut the tuna into dice (I prefer "chunkier" dice of about 1/2" inch each) and toss into the oil-spice-citrus mix. Add the scallions, and mix well. Cut the avocados in half, remove the seed, and peel. Cut the avocados into dice to match the size of your tuna dice. Carefully mix the avocado into the tuna mixture. Add the toasted sesame seeds, and season to taste. Allow the mixture to sit in the refrigerator for an hour for the flavors to blend. Serve on a bed of your julienned vegetables.

- Serve a red or white wine (rose) of fairly fruity character or a Sauvignon Blanc or a top Cotes du Rhone would be fine.

347. Tuna With Peppercorn Sauce Recipe

Serving: 4 | Prep: | Cook: 10mins | Ready in:

Ingredients

- 4 tuna steaks (about 1/2 lb. each)
- 1/4 teaspoon salt
- freshly ground black pepper
- 1 tablespoon olive oil -- divided
- 1 shallot -- minced
- 3/4 cup dry white wine
- 1 cup chicken broth or fish broth
- 1/2 cup heavy cream
- 1 tablespoon freeze-dried or brine-cured green peppercorns -- crushed or chopped
- 1 tbs chopped shallots is an option

Direction

- I like my tuna grilled (outside) and it is a meal that is worth the time.
- Sprinkle tuna with salt and pepper. Heat 2 teaspoons oil in a grill pan over medium heat for 1 minute. Add tuna and grill until almost cooked through, about 3 minutes per side. Transfer fish to a platter and cover with foil to keep warm.
- In a large nonstick skillet, heat remaining oil over medium heat. Add shallot and cook, stirring for 30 seconds. Add wine and cook until reduced to 1/4 cup, about 5 minutes. Add broth and cook until mixture reduces to 1 cup, about 5 minutes more.
- Pour in heavy cream and continue cooking until liquid is reduced again to 1 cup. Stir in peppercorns and juice that has accumulated from fish. Pour sauce over fish and serve immediately. You can garnish with a few of the peppercorns on the Tuna, but grill marks would look nice by themselves, from the outside grill.

348. Tuna In A Rich Tomato And Onion Sauce Recipe

Serving: 2 | Prep: | Cook: 20mins | Ready in:

Ingredients

- 1 1/2 lb tuna steaks (1 inch thick)
- 2 tb lemon juice
- 1 ts salt
- 1 ts ground turmeric
- vegetable oil
- 1/2 c flour
- 1/4 ts black pepper
- 4 tb vegetable oil
- 2 ts sugar
- 1 lg onion; finely chopped
- 1 tb ginger root; fresh grated
- 1 tb garlic; crushed
- 1 ts ground coriander
- 1 ts hot chile powder
- 8 oz canned diced tomatoes
- 1 1/4 c warm water
- 2 tb coriander; fresh chopped
- boiled rice

Direction

- Cut the fish into 3 inch pieces and put into a large bowl. Add the lemon juice and sprinkle with half the salt and half the turmeric. Mix gently with your fingertips and set aside for 15 minutes.
- Pour enough oil into a 9 inch frying pan to cover the base to a depth of 1/2 inch and heat over a medium setting. Mix the flour and pepper and dust the fish in the seasoned flour. Add to the oil in a single layer and fry until browned on both sides and a light crust has formed. Drain on kitchen paper.

- In a large pan, heat 4 tablespoon oil. When the oil is hot, but not smoking, add the sugar and let it caramelize. As soon as the sugar is brown, add the onion, ginger and garlic, and fry for 7-8 minutes, until just beginning to color. Stir regularly.
- Add the ground coriander, chili powder and the remaining turmeric. Stir fry for about 30 seconds and add the tomatoes. Cook until the tomatoes are mushy and the oil separates from the spice paste, stirring regularly.
- Pour the warm water and remaining salt into the pan, and bring to the boil. Carefully add the fried fish, reduce the heat to low and simmer, uncovered, for 5 to 6 minutes. Transfer to a serving dish and garnish with the coriander leaves. Serve over plain boiled rice.
- Note: This is an Eastern Indian, onion-rich dish, known as kalia in Bengal. A firm-fleshed fish is essential. Tuna works very nicely.

349. Under The Sea Seafood Casserole Recipe

Serving: 6 | Prep: | Cook: 30mins | Ready in:

Ingredients

- 2 tbsp butter
- 1tbsp olive oil
- 1 tbsp minced garlic
- 1 lbs firm flesh fish, such as ocean perch, catfish, etc - cubed
- 1 lbs medium shrimp, pealed and de-veined
- 1/2 lbs medium size scallop (fresh or thawed)
- 1/2 pound craw fish tail meat (fresh or thawed) - optional
- 1 lbs bag of frozen chopped spinach - thawed
- 1/2 green bell pepper, cored and sliced
- 1 tbsp dry tarragon
- 2 tbsp parsley flakes
- 1/2 lemon
- 1/2 tbsp kosher salt
- 2 tbsp Cajun/creole seasoning
- 1/2 tsp lemon pepper
- 1/2 tsp red pepper flakes
- 1 cup heavy cream

Direction

- Cube fish and sprinkle Cajun spice all over it.
- Slice bell pepper and thaw spinach according to the instructions on the package
- Heat oil and butter over medium heat
- Roast garlic until golden and fragrant
- Fold in all of the seafood and sauté for 5-6 minutes
- Add lemon juice, salt and all herbs and spices
- Add spinach and bell pepper
- Sauté over medium heat until all liquid is gone
- Add cream, heat through

350. Vera Cruz Red Snapper Recipe

Serving: 2 | Prep: | Cook: 15mins | Ready in:

Ingredients

- 2 pounds red snapper fillets
- juice of 1 lime
- 1 teaspoon salt
- 2 tablespoons olive oil
- 1 medium white onion chopped
- 1 bell pepper julienned
- 1 tablespoon garlic chopped
- 2 medium tomatoes chopped
- 1/4 cup green olives sliced
- 1 tablespoon capers
- 2 pickled jalapeno peppers

Direction

- Preheat oven to 450.
- Sprinkle fish with lime juice and salt.
- Set aside.
- Sauté onion, bell pepper, garlic and tomatoes in oil until softened.

- Simmer sauce until most of liquid is evaporated.
- Place fish in baking dish then top with sauce, olives, capers and chili peppers.
- Cover with foil and bake 15 minutes.

351. Vodka Martini Smoked Salmon Recipe

Serving: 8 | Prep: | Cook: 120mins | Ready in:

Ingredients

- 1 salmon, cleaned (about 3-4 pounds)
- 6 sprigs fresh dill
- 1/4 cup lemon juice
- 1/4 cup vodka
- 1/4 cup vermouth
- 3 tablespoons butter, melted
- 1 tablespoon horseradish
- 2 cloves garlic, minced
- 1 lemon, sliced
- 1/2 teaspoon hot sauce
- Preparation:
- Prepare charcoal grill for indirect cooking over hickory or alder wood chips.
- Wash salmon and pat dry. Fill with dill and lemon slices and set fish aside. Place remaining ingredients in small saucepan and bring to a boil. Remove from heat and set mixture aside.
- Lay salmon on a large piece of aluminum foil. Close three of the sides, pour in basting sauce, and fold over fourth edge. Place salmon on grill over a drip pan and allow to cook on low heat (about 225 degrees F.) for 1 hour. Open one side of the foil and let salmon cook for an additional hour.

Direction

- Prepare charcoal grill for indirect cooking over hickory or alder wood chips.
- Wash salmon and pat dry.
- Fill with dill and lemon slices and set fish aside.
- Place remaining ingredients in small saucepan and bring to a boil. Remove from heat and set mixture aside.
- Lay salmon on a large piece of aluminum foil.
- Close three of the sides, pour in basting sauce, and fold over fourth edge.
- Place salmon on grill over a drip pan and allow to cook on low heat (about 225 degrees F.) for 1 hour.
- Open one side of the foil and let salmon cook for an additional hour.

352. WRAPPED FARM RAISED CATFISH WITH CREAM CHEESE STUFFING Recipe

Serving: 4 | Prep: | Cook: 25mins | Ready in:

Ingredients

- 4 (6-8 oz.) farm-raised catfish fillets,fresh or frozen
- 1/2 teaspoon salt
- 1/4 teaspoon pepper
- 1 teaspoon lemon juice
- 1 cup fresh bread crumbs
- 3 tablespoons cream cheese
- 1 tablespoon lemon juice
- 1 tablespoon chopped celery
- 1 tablespoon chopped onion
- 1 teaspoon dried parsley
- 1 teaspoon ground thyme
- 1/2 teaspoon salt
- 1/4 teaspoon pepper
- 8 slices bacon
- lemon slices
- pimiento strips

Direction

- Thaw fish, if frozen. Season with 1/2 teaspoon salt and 1/4 teaspoon pepper. Sprinkle fish with 1 teaspoon lemon juice.
- Combine bread crumbs, cream cheese, 1 teaspoon lemon juice, celery, onion, parsley, thyme, 1/2 teaspoon salt, and 1/4 teaspoon pepper. Divide stuffing into 4portions. Place 1 portion of stuffing at one end of each fillet. Roll fish around stuffing.
- Fry bacon until cooked, but not crisp. Wrap 2 slices of bacon around each fillet; secure with a toothpick.
- Place fish rolls in a lightly greased baking dish. Bake in a moderate oven at 350 degrees for 15 - 20 minutes or until fish flakes easily when tested with a fork. Remove toothpicks before serving. Garnish with lemon slices and pimiento strips.

353. Walnut Crusted Halibut With Honey Soy Sauce Recipe

Serving: 4 | Prep: | Cook: 10mins | Ready in:

Ingredients

- 1 1/2 cups California walnuts, toasted
- 4 -6 oz Alaskan halibut filets
- 2 eggs lightly beaten with 1 tablespoon water
- 1/4 cup flour
- 1 tablespoon olive oil, light
- 1/3 cup soy sauce
- 2 cups clover honey
- Pinch of salt and pepper

Direction

- Pre-heat the oven to 375°F.
- Chop the walnuts.
- Stir a pinch of salt and pepper into the flour and reserve in a shallow dish.
- Whisk together the honey and soy sauce and reserve.
- Dip the halibut filets in the flour, coating thoroughly and shaking gently to remove any excess. Next dip them in the egg wash, draining off any excess, and immediately roll in the walnuts to coat. Reserve for 5 minutes to allow the coating to "set."
- Heat the olive oil in a sauté pan large enough to hold the filets and add the fish. Cook on one side until golden brown, flip carefully and finish in the oven for 5 minutes, or until cooked through.
- Arrange on a plate and drizzle with the reserved sauce.
- This is a The Cutting Horse Restaurant recipe.

354. Walnut Ginger Salmon Recipe

Serving: 4 | Prep: | Cook: 9mins | Ready in:

Ingredients

- 1 Tbs brown sugar
- 1 Tbs Dijon mustard
- 1 Tbs soy sauce
- 1 tsp ground ginger
- 4 skinless salmon fillets(4 oz. ea)
- 1/4 c walnuts

Direction

- In large re-sealable plastic bag, combine brown sugar, mustard, soy sauce and ginger; add the salmon. Seal bag and turn to coat; refrigerate for 30 mins, turning occasionally.
- Drain and discard marinade. Place salmon on foil-lined baking sheet coated with cooking spray. Broil 4-6" from the heat or till fish flakes easily with a fork, sprinkling with walnuts during the last 2 mins of cooking time.

355. Wasabi Pea Crusted Tuna Recipe

Serving: 4 | Prep: | Cook: 10mins | Ready in:

Ingredients

- 2 fresh tuna steaks, 1" thick (20 - 24 oz total)
- 5 oz wasabi peas
- 1 egg
- 1 C milk
- 1 C flour
- salt
- canola or other flavorless oil

Direction

- Cut each steak in half. Wash and dry them well and then wrap tightly in plastic wrap. Place in the freezer for about 45 minutes. Whisk the egg and the milk together. Crush the peas with a mortar and pestle until they have the consistency of very coarse salt. Unwrap and roll each piece of tuna in the flour, then dip them in the egg/milk mixture and then roll them in the crushed peas. Place on a plate and allow to rest for 10 minutes. Meanwhile, preheat a heavy cast-iron frying pan on low heat. After the resting-period is over, turn the heat to high and add about 3 tablespoons of oil to the pan. Allow to heat for about a minute and then add the fish pieces. With the heat on high, sauté the fish 1 minute on each side, including the edges. Remove and slice into one inch portions. Serve with soy sauce, shaved ginger and wasabi. Awesome!

356. West Coast Garlic Salmon Recipe

Serving: 4 | Prep: | Cook: 8mins | Ready in:

Ingredients

- 4 large salmon steaks
- 3 tablespoons butter melted
- 3 tablespoons peanut oil
- 2 tablespoons fresh lemon juice
- 2 tablespoons fresh minced garlic
- 1 teaspoon fresh tarragon minced
- 1/4 teaspoon grated lemon peel
- 1/8 teaspoon red pepper flakes
- 1 teaspoon salt
- 2 teaspoons freshly ground black pepper
- lemon wedges

Direction

- Combine butter, oil, lemon juice, tarragon, lemon peel and pepper flakes to make a marinade.
- Place salmon and broiler and brush with half the marinade.
- Broil under pre-heated broiler 2 inches from heat for 4 minutes.
- Turn and brush with remaining marinade then broil until fish flakes about 4 more minutes.
- Season with salt and pepper.
- Serve immediately with lemon wedges.

357. White Wine Salmon Corn Cakes Dated 1966 Recipe

Serving: 8 | Prep: | Cook: 15mins | Ready in:

Ingredients

- 2 cups water
- 1 cup dry white wine
- 1 bay leaf
- 4 whole peppercorns
- 2 parsley sprigs
- 5 celery leaves
- 2 salmon steaks
- 1 cup fresh corn kernels cooked
- 1/2 cup finely chopped shallots
- 1/2 cup finely diced red bell pepper
- 1/2 cup finely diced celery

- 1/4 cup chopped fresh cilantro leaves
- 1/2 cup plain yogurt drained
- 1/2 cup mayonnaise
- 1/2 teaspoon spicy mustard
- 1/2 teaspoon Tabasco sauce
- 1/4 teaspoon granulated salt
- 1/2 teaspoon freshly ground black pepper
- 1 egg plus 1 egg white lightly beaten
- 1-1/2 cups cracker crumbs
- 4 tablespoons olive oil

Direction

- Combine water, wine, bay leaf, peppercorns, parsley and celery leaves in shallow pan.
- Slowly bring to a boil then reduce to a simmer and add salmon steaks.
- Simmer until salmon is just cooked through then remove with slotted spatula.
- Drain and cool slightly then flake salmon into a bowl.
- Add corn, shallots, red pepper, celery and cilantro then fold together gently with rubber spatula.
- Combine yogurt, mayonnaise, mustard and Tabasco then fold into salmon mixture.
- Season with salt and pepper then gently fold egg, whites and 1/4 cup crumbs into salmon mix.
- Form into 8 large patties then lay some crumbs on a plate and coat patties on both sides.
- Refrigerate covered for up to 1 hour then heat 2 tablespoons oil in skillet over medium heat.
- Cook salmon corncakes a few at a time until golden about 3 minutes per side.
- Add more oil to skillet as needed.

358. Wild Pacific Salmon With Creamy Avocado Sauce Recipe

Serving: 6 | Prep: | Cook: 12mins | Ready in:

Ingredients

- 6 Wild Pacific salmon fillets (6 oz. each), about 1" thick
- 1/2 large avocado, peeled, pitted, and quartered
- 1/4 fat-free sour cream
- 1 Tbl. reduced-fat or light mayonnaise
- 1 tsp. lemon juice
- 1 clove garlic, minced
- 1/4 tsp. Hot-pepper sauce
- 1/4 tsp. salt
- 1/4 tsp. black pepper

Direction

- Place salmon fillets, skin side down, on foil-lined baking sheet. Coat fish with cooking spray (Olive Oil Spray) and season with salt and pepper.
- Preheat broiler. Cook salmon 10 to 12 minutes or until fish is opaque.
- While fish is cooking, combine avocado, sour cream, mayonnaise, lemon juice, garlic, hot-pepper sauce, Worcestershire sauce, salt, and pepper in a food processor. Process, scraping down bowl occasionally, until mixture is creamy and smooth.
- Serve dollop of sauce next to (or across the top of) salmon fillet.

359. Zesty Salmon Burgers Recipe

Serving: 2 | Prep: | Cook: 15mins | Ready in:

Ingredients

- 1 egg
- 1/4c dry bread crumbs
- 2 Tbs fine chopped onion
- 2 Tbs mayonaisse
- 11/2 to 3 tsp prepared horseradish
- 11/2 tsp diced pimientos
- 1/8 tsp salt
- dash pepper

- 1 pouch (7.1 oz.) boneless skinless pink salmon,drained

Direction

- In a small bowl, combine first 8 ingredients. Add salmon, mix well.
- Shape into 2 patties. On grill, brushed with oil, grill burgers at med heat for 5 to 6 mins on each side or till browned.
- Serve on rolls with lettuce.

360. Fried Tilapia With Thai Sauce Recipe

Serving: 2 | Prep: | Cook: 20mins | Ready in:

Ingredients

- 1 fresh tilapia
- 1 tbs of soy sauce
- 2 minced garlic
- 1 chilli, finely chopped
- juice of 1 lemon
- 5 tbs of thai sweet chilli sauce
- 2 tbs of chopped coriander

Direction

- Marinade fish with soy sauce and minced garlic.
- Deep fried until golden brown and crisp.
- My friend said that if you add a little salt in the oil, your fish won't stick to the wok.
- Mix chili sauce with lemon juice chili and coriander.
- Pour over fish, serve.

361. Indonesian Chilli Fish Recipe

Serving: 6 | Prep: | Cook: 30mins | Ready in:

Ingredients

- 2 tilapia or grouper or other small white flesh fish
- oil for frying
- 3 cloves garlic
- 2 shallots or half of an onion
- 4 chilli pepper
- 1 tbs salt
- 1/2 tbs sugar
- 2 cups of water
- pinch of white pepper
- ground coriander seed powder
- 200 ml coconut milk

Direction

- Deep fry the tilapia until golden brown on both sides.
- Using a mortar and pestle, bash garlic, shallots and chili and salt into a fine paste (or just finely slice them)
- Using a little oil, sauté this paste with low heat until fragrant; add water coconut milk and the rest of the ingredients; cook until the sauce is thickened.
- Taste, it should be rich, hot, spicy and not sweet (sugar is only to balance the flavor not to make it sweet); if it's not salty enough you can add a little more salt.

362. Sizzling Salmon Recipe

Serving: 2 | Prep: | Cook: 10mins | Ready in:

Ingredients

- 2 skinless and boneless fillets of salmon
- for the marinade:
- 1 and 1/2 tsp ginger paste
- 1 and 1/2 tsp garlic paste
- 1 tsp cumin powder
- 1 tsp corriander powder
- 1/2 tsp garam masala(optional)
- 1/2 tsp red chilli powder

- lemon juice(1 large lemon)
- salt to taste
- for pan frying:
- 1 tbsp cooking oil

Direction

- Mix all ingredients, except oil, in a bowl and marinade the salmon fillets in it for 15 mins.
- Take the oil in a non-stick frying pan.
- Heat the pan on medium flame.
- Pan-fry the marinated fillets from all sides for 10 mins or till the fillets change color.
- Serve hot on a bed of steamed rice or green salad.
- Goes well with a glass of white wine.
- Can be alternatively grilled in the oven (on medium for 5 mins on each side) or barbequed.

363. Stuffed Whole Flounder Recipe

Serving: 2 | Prep: | Cook: 37mins | Ready in:

Ingredients

- 1 small flounder cleaned & butterflied
- 1/2 cup flakey crab meat
- 1/4 cup small shrimp shelled & deviened (raw salad shrimp)
- 1 cup herbed stuffing (bagged dry)
- 1 tbls. minced onion
- 1/2 tbls. minced green bell pepper
- 1 tsp. old bay
- 1/4 cup mayonaise
- salt &pepper
- butter

Direction

- In mixing bowl, combine all ingredients until smooth workable stuffing forms; salt & pepper to taste. Reserve butter & melt (1/4 stick +/-). Stuff flounder under each pouch and pile in middle cavity. Pour some of butter over entire fish and stuffing. Bake at 400 degrees in well-buttered pan until stuffing is done golden brown color; garnish with lemon slices and parsley. Serve.

364. Sweet Ginger Mahi Mahi Recipe

Serving: 2 | Prep: | Cook: 10mins | Ready in:

Ingredients

- 2 8 oz mahi mahi fillets
- 3 tbsp honey (or maple syrup)
- 3 tbsp soy sauce
- 3 tbsp balsamic vinegar
- 1 tsp grated fresh ginger root
- 1 clove garllic, crushed
- 4 tsp olive oil

Direction

- Combine all ingredients except fish in a large freezer bag
- Add fish; turn to coat and refrigerate for 20 min
- Heat grill to Medium heat and brush lightly with olive oil
- Remove fillets from marinade (reserve liquid) and grill for 10-12 min, turning once-until fish flakes with a fork.
- Pour reserved marinade into a small skillet and heat over medium flame until mixture reduces to a thick glaze, 2-3 minutes
- Spoon glaze over fish and serve immediately
- Delicious!

365. ~ Swim ~ Recipe

Serving: 2 | Prep: | Cook: | Ready in:

Ingredients

- 4 Rainbow trout...butterflied,dehead,and pin bones removed
- sea salt and Fresh Gind pepper
- 5 oz. Boursin...leave out to take the chill off, and soften ever so slightly
- 1/2 Cup roasted red peppers,cut in thin strips
- 2 1/2 Cups baby spinach leaves,given a shower and dried
- 3 Tablespoons olive oil
- 2 Tablespoon Farm Fresh Butter

Direction

- Season the cavity inside of each Trout with salt and pepper.
- Blend the Boursin, Red Pepper, and Baby Spinach; season with sea salt and pepper...mix thoroughly.
- Place one fourth of the stuffing inside each Trout.
- Very carefully fold one side of the Trout to the other side, encasing the stuffing between the two halves.
- Place the oil and butter in fry pan over a medium heat...when butter stops foaming, place Trout in pan skin side down.
- Sear about 4 minutes or until skin is crisp.
- Flip Trout and crisp the other side as well.
- Remove from the pan...and as if that's not enough meet the heat...place on greased baking sheet and bake in a 350 degree oven for about 10 minutes, or until cooked through.
- Note: Serve with a very nice well-oaked Chardonnay Wine, or a Sancerre.
- ~ I don't care what they say...Don't go down with the ship...You are master of your fate...You are Captain of you own vessel.
- Melt that iceberg...or...SWIM...FISHY...SWIM...As if your life depended on it ~

Index

A

B

C

D

E

F

G

H

J

K

L

M

N

O

P

R

S

Conclusion

Thank you again for downloading this book!

I hope you enjoyed reading about my book!

If you enjoyed this book, please take the time to share your thoughts and post a review on Amazon. It'd be greatly appreciated!

Write me an honest review about the book – I truly value your opinion and thoughts and I will incorporate them into my next book, which is already underway.

Thank you!

If you have any questions, **feel free to contact at:** *author@cuminrecipes.com*

Jennifer Wilson

cuminrecipes.com